FATTY LIVER DIET COOKBOOK

Your Comprehensive Blueprint to Detoxify, Energize, and Revitalize Your Liver.

Discover Irresistible Recipes and Leverage a Tailored 12-Week Meal Plan for Optimal Liver Health.

OLIVIA GREENLEAF

1 Introduction

1.1 Understanding Fatty Liver Disease

Fatty liver disease isn't just a medical term; for many, it's a lived reality. Also known as hepatic steatosis, it's what happens when your liver becomes a reluctant storage unit for excess fats. Sure, a little fat is par for the course, as normal as having a junk drawer in your kitchen. But when that drawer starts to overflow, blocking the rest of your life? Well, then we're looking at complications that could easily escalate.

The world of fatty liver disease has two main districts, so to speak: one where the culprit is alcohol and another where it's anything but. The medical community labels them as alcoholic fatty liver disease (AFLD) and non-alcoholic fatty liver disease (NAFLD). AFLD is a fairly straightforward tale—a love affair with booze gone awry. NAFLD, on the other hand, is our focus today. Think of it as a complicated web woven by lifestyle choices—like a diet straight out of a fast-food menu, an aversion to exercise, or the extra pounds that sneak up on you over the years.

Yet, even within NAFLD's murky depths, there are layers. You could have a simple fatty liver, also known as steatosis, which is mostly a quiet tenant. It stays put, takes up some room, but generally doesn't throw wild parties that disrupt the neighborhood. In other words, it's typically symptom-free and won't drastically shorten your lifespan. But then there's its more menacing sibling, non-alcoholic steatohepatitis or NASH. NASH doesn't just sit around; it starts a fire in the form of inflammation and liver damage. Over time, this can pave the way for fibrosis, a type of tissue scarring that's about as welcome as weeds in a garden, ultimately obstructing the liver's crucial functions. And if that's not dire enough, untreated NASH could even metamorphose into liver cirrhosis or cancer, the equivalent of a quiet street turning into a disaster zone.

Alarmingly, this isn't some rare, isolated issue. A quarter of the world's population is estimated to have NAFLD. Its prevalence is spreading, a somber shadow that grows alongside rising obesity and type 2 diabetes rates. Kids aren't immune either; it's a family affair affecting all ages. Dig a little deeper, and you'll find that about one in five individuals with NAFLD also has the more serious NASH.

One of the most insidious aspects of fatty liver disease is its ability to hide in plain sight. It's the wallflower at the party, the spy in a thriller novel—easy to overlook. No symptoms may manifest in the early stages, meaning you could share your life with this silent partner for years, blissfully ignorant of its presence. Hence, it's paramount to know your enemies—obesity, high levels of cholesterol, metabolic syndrome, type 2 diabetes, and insulin resistance are the usual suspects. Yet, remember, even seemingly 'healthy' people, without these obvious risk factors, aren't safe. It's not just the usual suspects that are problematic; lifestyle choices like poor diet, lack of physical activity, and high stress are the less-noticeable termites

1

eating away at your health.

If this all seems like an overwhelming labyrinth of issues, take heart: understanding fatty liver disease is your first torch in a dark cave. As daunting as it might seem, the flicker of hope is that lifestyle and dietary changes can often reverse NAFLD. Consider this book your roadmap to navigating out of this mess. It's not just information; it's your guide to retaking your health, reclaiming your life, and rerouting your destiny.

1.2 The Role of Diet in Managing and Reversing Fatty Liver

The foods you eat aren't just a matter of personal taste; they are foundational bricks in the architecture of your well-being. Imagine your liver as a diligent worker in the recycling center of your body, sorting and breaking down fats and toxins. When you flood that worker with saturated fats, artificial ingredients, and sugar, it's akin to dumping a truckload of plastic waste into a recycling facility designed for paper; the system gets clogged, and the operations falter. Over time, this may lead to your liver filling with fats, kicking off a chain of events that includes inflammation and, ultimately, liver damage.

Now, picture your kitchen as the anti-inflammatory headquarters, where you wage a daily war on fatty liver. No, you don't need to adopt an ascetic, joyless eating pattern; rather, think of it as an artistic endeavor in making mindful choices that are easy on your liver. You're not putting your cravings under a lifelong curfew; you're building a roadmap to lifelong health. Here's what a liver-friendly terrain looks like:

At the top of the blacklist are sugars and processed foods. Imagine these as the toxic friends you need to distance yourself from. They come in appealing packages—cakes, white bread, fast food—but all they really offer is a clutter of unhealthy fats, sugar, and additives that fire up inflammation in your liver. Next, elevate your fiber game. Whole grains, leafy greens, fruits, and legumes are the infantry in this fight— armed with antioxidants, they not only keep blood sugar levels in check but also throw a counterpunch at liver inflammation.

Now, let's talk fats, but the good kind—think of them as the cherished members of your squad. Avocados, olive oil, and fatty fish like salmon serve to temper the inflammation. Meanwhile, your liver needs proteins as its building blocks. Go for the good stuff—lean poultry, fish, plant-based proteins like beans and lentils, and even tofu are your go-to repair kits for liver cells.

Amid all this, remember that water is your best friend. Just as plants need water to thrive, your liver requires it to flush out toxins and keep the system running smoothly.

And if you're searching for a compass to guide you through this journey, look no further than the Mediterranean diet. Picture a meal plan as scenic and soothing as a Mediterranean beach at sunset. Studies show that this diet—a pageant of fruits, veggies, lean proteins, and healthy fats—acts like a healing balm on liver fat and inflammation.

Of course, your culinary strategy is but one part of a broader lifestyle overhaul. Regular exercise, alcohol abstinence, and mindful medication are essential auxiliary troops in this mission. The objective isn't a quick-fix diet but a sea change in how you relate to food. A sustainable transformation, if you will. Don't forget—these dietary shifts are like individual brushstrokes in a larger masterpiece. Each contributes not just to a rejuvenated liver but to an empowered, healthier you. There are additional dividends too: reduced risk of heart disease and diabetes, uplifted moods, and even elevated energy levels. Taking control of fatty liver through diet isn't a trek on an unmarked path. It's a navigable journey, especially when you've got the right map and compass. This book aims to be your guide, offering concrete steps, scientific foundations, and even a recipe or two, turning the task of reclaiming your liver health from an uphill battle to a scenic, enlightening journey.

1.3 The Importance of Exercise and Healthy Lifestyle Changes

When it comes to battling fatty liver disease, diet isn't the only weapon in your arsenal. Exercise is another crucial element—think of it as your second line of defense. But this isn't just about liver health. Engaging in regular physical activity carries a cascade of benefits that spill over into various realms of your well-being. Exercise isn't just a luxury; it's a necessity in combating this pervasive ailment.

What's so magical about moving your body? First off, exercise helps keep your insulin levels in check. This is vital because a condition like fatty liver often has a sinister accomplice: insulin resistance. That's not all. Physical activity also helps you lose weight, which directly reduces the fatty deposits in your liver. And as if that's not enough, exercise also lowers inflammation and gives your metabolism a much-needed boost. All of these factors contribute to a healthier liver and, by extension, a healthier you.

You might be thinking, "Do I need to run a marathon or live in the gym?" Not at all. The good news is, even moderate forms of exercise can make a huge difference. Whether it's a brisk walk in the park, a leisurely cycle through the neighborhood, or a swim in the local pool, what counts is getting your heart rate up. The general recommendation is at least 150 minutes of moderate-intensity or 75 minutes of vigorous-intensity exercise every week. And if you're just stepping onto the fitness bandwagon, start slow—your body will thank you for the gradual introduction.

Yet, there's more to this journey than just diet and exercise. Other lifestyle choices also hold significant sway over your liver's health. Losing weight, for instance, is one of the best things you can do. In fact, shedding just 5-10% of your total body weight can often result in marked improvements in liver function. Alcohol is another major player. Even if alcohol didn't cause your liver problems, cutting back—or cutting it out entirely—will only help your liver heal.

Don't overlook the subtler factors, like toxins and sleep. Medications you don't really need or environmental pollutants could be sneakily undermining your liver health. Be vigilant about what you expose yourself to. Then there's sleep. A good night's sleep is about more than just feeling rested; it's a cornerstone of overall health and well-being. Skimping on sleep could actually increase your risk of developing fatty liver disease.

Stress is another shadowy contributor to fatty liver and a host of other health issues. To keep it at bay, consider integrating practices like meditation, yoga, or mindfulness into your daily routine. These tools can help manage stress, making your path to liver health a bit smoother.

Look, there are going to be bumps on the road to a healthier liver and a healthier you. It's perfectly normal to hit a few snags along the way. The key is persistence and the understanding that even small, sustainable changes can make a significant impact on your health. Luckily, you don't have to go it alone. This book serves as a reliable companion, offering you not just facts but practical advice to guide you on this transformative journey towards wellness.

1.4 How to Use This Book

Think of this book as your personal road map to a healthier liver and a more fulfilling life. It's designed to meet you wherever you are on your journey, whether you're just coming to grips with a fatty liver diagnosis or you're knee-deep in the recovery process. The layout? User-friendly. The goal? To adapt to your unique life circumstances.

We kick things off with the ABCs of fatty liver disease—what triggers it, why it's a big deal, and what you can do to treat it. We aim to arm you with the necessary knowledge, to lay the groundwork for everything that follows. That being said, let's be clear: This book is a treasure trove of insights, but it's not a substitute for personalized medical guidance. Make sure you keep your healthcare provider in the loop.

Next, we pivot to the kitchen, the battlefield where much of your liver's fate will be determined. The chapters on diet are structured to make the information easy to digest (pun intended). We'll discuss what to pile on your plate and what to banish from your pantry, explaining the 'whys' along the way. And because navigating a grocery store can feel like navigating a minefield, we've got you covered with a rundown of key nutrients and their superpowers.

Now, let's talk food—delicious, nourishing, home-cooked food. We're serving up 120 mouth-watering recipes that span breakfast, lunch, dinner, snacks, and yes, even beverages. Each recipe comes complete with the time you'll need to prep and cook, the ingredients you'll use, and a step-by-step guide to putting it all together. They're packed with nutrients, easy on the skill level, and as tasty as they are health-promoting. Plus, each recipe comes with a full nutritional breakdown, letting you keep tabs on macronutrients.

But hey, we get it—eating for your liver shouldn't mean sidelining your taste buds or those of your loved ones. That's why these recipes aim for universal deliciousness. They're meals you'll look forward to, meals that'll make everyone at the table happy.

Meal planning? We've made it a no-brainer with a 30-day meal plan tailored to tickle your taste buds and set you on the path to liver recovery. Feel free to treat it as a suggestion, not a script; you're welcome to play culinary DJ, mixing and matching to suit your own preferences and needs.

Yet, what you eat is just part of the equation. That's why we dive deep into the role of exercise and lifestyle changes—things like getting active and making other holistic adjustments to your daily routine. We've included practical tips and strategies to make these changes stick, all aimed at rounding out your approach to liver health.

Taking it slow? That's totally fine. Rome wasn't built in a day and neither is a healthier you. The book is here whenever you need a reference, a guide, or even a dose of inspiration.

In the end, this book isn't just about improving your liver; it's about enhancing your overall quality of life. Whether you're here for the deep dive into fatty liver disease, the culinary adventure, or the 30-day meal plan, remember that every page you turn and every step you take brings you closer to a better, healthier version of yourself. Cheers to the journey ahead!

2 The Fundamentals

2.1 Understanding Nutrition and Your Liver

The liver: it's not just another organ. This powerhouse is essentially the body's chemistry lab, and it's constantly hard at work. From producing bile that aids digestion, to breaking down an array of nutrients, to detoxifying harmful substances, the liver's roles are both numerous and vital. And guess what? What you eat plays a starring role in how well this vital organ functions.

Think of your liver as a highly sensitive processing plant. It's the first stop for everything you ingest, which makes your diet a critical factor for its health. Eating right isn't just a fad; it can ward off and even reverse liver conditions, like non-alcoholic fatty liver disease, commonly known as NAFLD.

But what does "eating right" entail, exactly? For starters, let's talk macronutrients: carbohydrates, proteins, and fats. Carbs aren't the enemy; it's the type of carbs that matter. The liver thrives on complex carbs found in whole grains, fruits, and vegetables. These not only fuel the liver but also come loaded with dietary fiber. This helps in more ways than one, like keeping blood sugar levels steady and reducing the risk of fatty deposits accumulating in the liver.

Proteins are another key player. The liver needs them for a variety of biochemical wizardry, including the synthesis of certain crucial proteins. So, what should be on your plate? Think lean meats, beans, nuts, seeds, and low-fat dairy—foods that are rich in protein but not in regret.

Fats, however, are a trickier game. Good fats like those found in avocados, nuts, and olive oil can be your liver's allies, aiding in hormone production and vitamin absorption. On the flip side, bad fats—the saturated and trans fats commonly found in fried and processed foods—can spell trouble. They can lead to fat accumulation in the liver, setting the stage for NAFLD.

Of course, the story doesn't end with macronutrients. Your liver also needs a supporting cast of micronutrients. Essential vitamins like B, E, and C, along with minerals like zinc and selenium, do more than just add alphabetic diversity; they serve functions ranging from detoxification to liver protection.

Water isn't just for quenching your thirst; it's crucial for your liver's detoxifying role. It's like giving your liver a helping hand in flushing out the nasties.

And while we're talking about things to ingest, let's touch on what to avoid. Alcohol, excessive salt and sugar, processed foods, and certain medications don't do your liver any favors. In fact, they're the bad crowd your liver should definitely avoid hanging out with.

So, let's sum it up: how you fuel your body has a direct and profound effect on your liver's health. Knowledge is power, and understanding the nutritional impact on your liver is the first step to making better dietary choices. Choices that ease the workload on your liver, allowing it to function at its best, which in turn leads to a healthier, happier you. After all, food can either be the most effective form of medicine or a ticking time bomb. The choice, as they say, is yours.

2.2 Foods to Embrace and Foods to Avoid

If you're aiming for a liver that's as fit as a fiddle, your diet is the cornerstone. Not only can the right foods keep your liver cruising smoothly, but they can also help flip the script on liver ailments, like the increasingly common non-alcoholic fatty liver disease (NAFLD). So what should you load up your shopping cart with, and what should you steer clear of? Let's dive in.

First up, let's talk about the heroes of a liver-friendly diet. Fruits and veggies, those nutritional all-stars, are jam-packed with vitamins, minerals, and fiber. And guess what? They're also a bonanza of antioxidants, which act like your liver's personal bodyguards. Want to diversify your nutrient portfolio? Make room for berries, papaya, avocados, bananas, and an assortment of leafy greens like spinach and kale.

Whole grains are another must-have. Think brown rice, oatmeal, quinoa, and anything that's made from whole grain. These guys are rich in complex carbs that fuel you, not to mention the dietary fiber that helps your digestive system hum along.

Then there are proteins. Yes, your liver loves them, but lean is the keyword here. Fish, lean meats, poultry, eggs—these are your liver's protein pals. Vegetarian? No worries. Beans, lentils, and tofu are fabulous plant-based options.

Healthy fats deserve a spot on your plate, too. Opt for those that are monounsaturated and polyunsaturated, like the fats in olive oil, avocados, and various nuts and seeds. These fats do a neat little trick: they lower the "bad" LDL cholesterol while giving the "good" HDL a boost. And if you're into seafood, fatty fish like salmon and mackerel are worth their weight in omega-3s.

Dairy can be a double-edged sword. While it provides essential calcium and vitamin D, it can also come with unnecessary fats. Your best bet? Go for low-fat or no-fat varieties. And if you're looking to spice things up, herbs and spices like turmeric, garlic, and ginger not only add zest to your meals but also come with bonus health benefits, including anti-inflammatory action.

Now, onto the no-go list. Sugar and refined carbs are your liver's nemesis. White bread, pasta, and those tempting pastries can result in a fatty liver over time. Saturated and trans fats, found lurking in fried and processed foods and fatty cuts of meat, are cholesterol culprits that your liver could do without.

While we're at it, let's not overlook salt. Sure, it perks up your food, but too much can send your blood pressure into the stratosphere and put additional stress on your liver. Last but definitely not least, alcohol is a known liver wrecker that can lead to cirrhosis and even liver cancer. If you've got liver issues, it's best to ditch the booze altogether.

In a nutshell, liver health isn't just about avoiding bad foods; it's about embracing the good ones. The key is balance. No one's saying you can't have a treat now and then, but making wise choices most of the time can work wonders not just for your liver, but for your whole body and mind. So next time you're about to chow down, remember: your liver is what it eats.

2.3 The Role of Fasting in Liver Health

Fasting is far from a new trend; it's an ancient practice, steeped in spiritual and religious traditions that stretch back thousands of years. In recent times, however, the scientific community has started to perk up its ears and examine the potential health gains of fasting, particularly where the liver is concerned.

Your liver isn't just an organ hanging out in your abdomen; it's a vital control center for your body's energy supply. When you eat more than you immediately need, your body stashes the extra glucose away as glycogen, mostly in the liver. During periods when you fast, the liver converts this glycogen back into energy, essentially performing metabolic magic. For people dealing with fatty liver issues, this process can be more than a little helpful, helping shed those excess fat deposits in the liver.

But the benefits don't stop there. Fasting sets off a cascade of cellular housekeeping known as autophagy. Think of it as your body's internal recycling program. Cells ditch their damaged or unnecessary parts, making room for healthier, more functional components. For your liver, this is like a rejuvenating spa treatment at the cellular level. Damaged cells get replaced with new, functional ones, bolstering your liver's overall performance.

When it comes to fasting methods, you've got options. A lot of people have hopped on the intermittent fasting bandwagon, toggling between periods of eating and not eating. You can fast daily within a specific 8-hour window or perhaps adopt a 5:2 model, where you eat normally for five days and then dramatically cut back on calories for two. Time-restricted feeding is another intriguing approach, where you only eat within a super-narrow 4- to 6-hour window each day. And let's not forget periodic fasting, which entails eating significantly less for a few days every several weeks or months.

Despite its virtues, fasting isn't a one-size-fits-all solution. If you're dealing with health conditions like diabetes, this isn't something to jump into without a chat with your doctor. And let's be clear: fasting is not a hall pass for eating junk food in your non-fasting hours. The benefits of fasting are best reaped when it's part of an overall health-conscious lifestyle that includes a balanced, nutritious diet.

In essence, fasting can serve as a robust tool in your liver health toolkit. It can work wonders on diminishing fat stores and encouraging the rejuvenation of liver cells. Yet, this should be integrated into a broader, more holistic approach to health, which includes regular exercise and balanced nutrition. And remember, it's wise to have a sit-down with a healthcare expert before making such a radical change to your eating patterns. Fasting can be a game-changer for your liver, but like anything else that's impactful, it needs to be done sensibly and responsibly.

2.4 Exercise Recommendations for Fatty Liver

Being told you have fatty liver disease can certainly be a jarring moment. It's one of those health conditions that suddenly shines a light on the life choices you've made, pushing you toward healthier habits. Among these, exercise is no minor player; it's a cornerstone of both managing and potentially rolling back the impacts of fatty liver disease.

Your liver is more than just another organ; it's your body's multi-tasker, tackling everything from detoxification to protein synthesis and creating essential digestive chemicals. When fat accumulates in this vital organ, as happens with fatty liver disease, these essential functions can take a hit. More often than not, the excess fat is a byproduct of poor dietary choices, insufficient physical activity, and the resulting weight gain.

So why does exercise matter? Even if the scale doesn't immediately reflect your efforts, physical activity does wonders for your liver by lowering the fat content within the liver cells. More broadly, regular exercise helps you manage your weight, which is vital in reducing fat both in your liver and your body as a whole.

Alright, so how should you go about this exercise thing? First off, consistency is your best friend. Aim for at least 75 to 150 minutes of moderate-intensity exercise per week. You could go for a brisk walk, hop on a bike, do a bit of swimming, or even engage in some high-intensity house chores. The point is to get moving. Secondly, don't underestimate the power of strength training. Incorporate it into your routine a couple of days a week to build muscle mass, which subsequently fires up your metabolism. If you're feeling adventurous, high-intensity interval training (HIIT) offers a more intense yet effective workout regime. For the rest of the day, simple changes like choosing stairs over elevators and parking at the far end of the lot can make a difference too. These are categorized as Non-Exercise Physical Activities (NEPA) and they contribute to your overall health. Yoga and Pilates might not directly aid in weight loss, but they can do wonders for your flexibility, balance, and mental well-being, which all indirectly support your health journey.

Here's a pro-tip: The exercise routine that will work best for you is the one you'll actually do. Choose activities you enjoy and if possible, recruit a buddy for mutual motivation and accountability. And don't forget, before jumping into a new exercise regimen, have a word with your healthcare provider. They can tailor your workout plan according to any underlying health conditions or constraints you may have.

To wrap it up, exercise isn't just beneficial for your liver; it's indispensable. A balanced blend of aerobic exercises, strength training, and even lifestyle changes can help lower liver fat and rejuvenate liver function. But don't treat exercise as a silver bullet. It needs to work in tandem with a balanced diet to really tackle fatty liver disease effectively. Exercise may be a pillar of liver health, but it's still part of a bigger, holistic approach to wellness.

3 Preparation Essentials

3.1 Kitchen Tools and Essentials for a Healthy Kitchen

Deciding to make healthier lifestyle choices often starts right in the heart of your home: the kitchen. A well-equipped kitchen can make all the difference when you're trying to prepare liver-friendly, nutritious meals. It not only streamlines the culinary process but also gives you the inspiration to experiment, have fun, and engage wholeheartedly in your health journey.

The first thing you'll want to check off your list? Quality cookware. Investing in sturdy pots, pans, and a baking sheet can be transformative. If you opt for non-stick versions, you'll find you need less oil, nudging your meals toward the healthier end of the spectrum. Look after them well, and they'll return the favor for years to come.

Don't underestimate the value of good cutting tools. A couple of sharp, quality knives—think a versatile chef's knife, a precision-oriented paring knife, and a serrated knife for all things crusty and tough—can revolutionize your food prep. And it goes without saying that a decent cutting board is non-negotiable.

As for gadgets? Consider a high-quality blender or food processor. Beyond smoothies, these workhorses are perfect for soups, sauces, and even liver-friendly spreads like hummus. Measuring tools are your next pit stop. A set of measuring cups and spoons along with a kitchen scale ensures that you're not playing fast and loose with recipe proportions.

Moving on to the basics, you'll want to have a collection of mixing bowls, various sizes at that. And for utensils? A spatula, a slotted spoon, and a set of tongs should cover most bases. If your life is a whirlwind of work meetings and errands, you might find a slow cooker or a pressure cooker to be your new best friend. Prepare your ingredients in the morning, and you'll walk home to a freshly cooked meal.

When it comes to healthy cooking methods, steamers and grill pans earn their keep. Steaming is a nutrient-conserving, fat-free way to cook, particularly suited for vegetables and fish. A grill pan not only brings out rich flavors but also helps drain off excess fat. And let's not forget storage! Opt for glass containers; they're sturdy, reusable, and transparent, which makes identifying leftovers a breeze.

In terms of pantry essentials, think of stocking up on lean proteins, an assortment of fruits and veggies, whole grains, and of course, spices and herbs for that extra zing. Healthy fats like avocados and olive oil are also beneficial. Let's not forget hydration—after all, it's vital for liver health. A good water filter ensures you're sipping the cleanest water possible.

No need to rush out and buy all of this in one fell swoop. Begin where you can, and gradually expand your toolkit. You're not just investing in kitchenware; you're investing in yourself, in your own health. In the grand scheme of things, that's more than worth the price of admission. Eating for liver health isn't about cutting things out; it's about embracing a wide palette of nutrient-rich foods. Get your kitchen ready for this adventure, and you'll find that it's not just your liver that's thriving—your entire approach to wellness will transform.

3.2 Understanding and Converting Measurements

Navigating the culinary landscape often feels like learning a new language, especially when you're staring down a laundry list of measurements that might as well be written in hieroglyphics. Yet, mastering this numerical jargon is far less intimidating than it appears at first glance.

First things first, the yardsticks you'll encounter most frequently in the kitchen revolve around either volume or weight. In the United States, you'll bump into a lineup of volume-based measurements— teaspoons, tablespoons, and cups, just to name a few. On the other side of the Atlantic and beyond, milliliters and liters are the order of the day. These units help measure liquid ingredients or those that can be easily poured.

However, when it comes to baking, weight trumps volume for accuracy. American recipes lean towards ounces and pounds, while the rest of the globe opts for grams and kilograms. Knowing how these units correspond is your first leg up in the world of conversion. For example, a tablespoon holds three teaspoons, a cup contains 16 tablespoons, and so on. In terms of weight, it's good to remember that one ounce is approximately 28.35 grams and a pound contains 16 ounces.

Simple multiplication and division will get you far in the conversion game. But if numbers make your eyes glaze over, fear not. There's an army of conversion charts and digital calculators ready to jump to your aid. Pro tip: Stick a printed conversion chart on your fridge or inside a kitchen cabinet. It's an old-school solution, but incredibly handy.

Imagine you stumble upon a recipe that demands a cup of all-purpose flour, but you're armed only with a scale that measures in grams. A quick glance at your conversion chart informs you that one cup of flour is equivalent to 125 grams. Problem solved, you just weigh the required amount. Be wary though; when dealing with dry ingredients like flour, conversions can get tricky due to factors like compaction. That's why many culinary pros advocate for weight over volume, especially in baking, where precision is key.

Temperature shouldn't be overlooked, either. If your oven talks in Fahrenheit and your recipe in Celsius, a quick formula or chart will bridge the gap. To convert Fahrenheit to Celsius, you use the formula $(°F - 32) \times 5/9 = °C$, and vice versa.

The intricacies of cooking measurements may seem daunting at first, but like any skill, it gets easier with practice and the right resources. And speaking of resources, the end of this book offers a chapter dedicated solely to conversion tables. Soon enough, you'll be flipping through any recipe like it's your native tongue.

3.3 Shopping List and Pantry Essentials

The old saying "Out of sight, out of mind" carries more truth than you might think, especially when it comes to managing a fatty liver diet. If your pantry is filled with the right foods, you're far more likely to stick to healthier choices. Think of your pantry as your first line of defense: what you stock in it sets the tone for what ends up on your plate.

First off, let's talk grains. Whole grains, to be specific. These nutritional powerhouses—like brown rice, whole grain bread, quinoa, and oats—are teeming with fiber that aids in digestion and weight management. These factors are indispensable when it comes to combating fatty liver disease. So when you're out shopping, whole grains should be at the top of your list.

Proteins, too, are crucial. They're the building blocks that help repair and maintain liver health. But not all proteins are created equal. Stick to lean options like chicken breast, turkey, and fish. For vegetarians or those looking to diversify, plant-based proteins such as lentils, chickpeas, and tofu are excellent substitutions.

Now, what about fruits and veggies? Aim to have them take up at least half the real estate on your plate every mealtime. They're the providers of essential vitamins and minerals and are also rich in antioxidants, which fight inflammation. Go for a colorful variety—leafy greens, berries, bell peppers, and sweet potatoes are all fantastic.

As for fats, you want to focus on the good guys: avocados, olives, nuts, and seeds. These fats not only help tamp down liver inflammation but also assist in absorbing vitamins like A, D, E, and K, which are fat-soluble. Moving to spices and herbs, flavor isn't their only strength. Many, like turmeric, have proven anti-inflammatory properties. Don't overlook ginger, garlic, and cinnamon, which also offer health benefits.

Dairy can be a bit of a minefield. The key here is to opt for low-fat or non-fat options that give you the calcium and protein you require, minus the excess fat and calories. And when it comes to beverages, keep it simple. Water should be your go-to, although green tea also earns high marks for its antioxidants. Steer clear of alcohol and sugary drinks; they're not doing your liver any favors.

When you're jotting down your shopping list, aim for fresh, minimally processed foods. Avoid items loaded with added sugars, sodium, and unhealthy fats. Always read labels; manufacturers are experts at sneaking in unhealthy additives and hidden sugars. To make things even easier, consider meal planning. It's a lifesaver for making sure you have what you need for the week, and it'll steer you clear of those unhealthy, last-minute food choices.

This book, by the way, is filled with a wealth of liver-friendly recipes aimed at setting you on the path to better health. The ultimate goal isn't to achieve dietary perfection, but to make incremental, sustainable changes you can live with long-term. Because, when it comes down to it, the journey to a healthier liver starts in your kitchen. With the right foods and the right tools, you're not just setting yourself up for success—you're already halfway there.

4 Breakfast Recipes

4.1 Avocado and Egg White Omelet

Preparation time: 10 minutes   **Cooking time:** 10 minutes   **Servings:** 1

Ingredients:

- 3 Egg Whites
- 1/2 Ripe Avocado, sliced
- 1/4 Cup Spinach, roughly chopped
- 1/4 Cup Tomatoes, diced
- Salt and Pepper to taste
- 1 Teaspoon Olive Oil

Directions:

1. Heat the olive oil over medium heat in a non-stick frying pan.
2. In a bowl, whisk the egg whites until frothy. Add a pinch of salt and pepper.
3. Pour the egg whites into the pan and let them cook undisturbed until they start to set around the edges, about 2-3 minutes.
4. Scatter the spinach and tomatoes evenly over half of the omelet. Let it cook for another minute.
5. Place the sliced avocado on top of the vegetables.
6. Carefully fold the other half of the omelet over the vegetables and avocado.
7. Let it cook for another 2-3 minutes until the omelet is fully set and the vegetables are heated through.
8. Use a spatula to slide the omelet onto a plate. Serve immediately.

Calories: 215   **Protein:** 14g   **Fat:** 15g   **Carbohydrates:** 7g

4.2 Overnight Chia Pudding with Almond Milk and Fresh Berries

Preparation time: 10 minutes   **Cooking time:** 8 hours (overnight)   **Servings:** 2

Ingredients:

- 1/4 Cup Chia Seeds
- 1 Cup Unsweetened Almond Milk
- 1 Teaspoon Pure Vanilla Extract
- 1-2 Tablespoons Pure Maple Syrup or Honey (optional)
- A Pinch of Salt
- 1 Cup Fresh Berries (strawberries, blueberries, raspberries, etc.)

Directions:

1. In a bowl or mason jar, mix together chia seeds, almond milk, vanilla extract, sweetener if using, and a pinch of salt.
2. Stir well to ensure there are no clumps of chia seeds. Let the mixture sit for 5 minutes, then stir again.
3. Cover the container and refrigerate overnight, or for at least 6-8 hours.
4. In the morning, give the chia pudding a good stir. It should have a thick and creamy consistency.
5. Top with fresh berries just before serving. You can also add other toppings like nuts or seeds if you like.

Calories: 200   **Protein:** 6g   **Fat:** 9g   **Carbohydrates:** 25g

4.3 Turmeric Smoothie with Banana, Spinach, and Flaxseeds

Preparation time: 10 minutes **Cooking time:** No cooking required **Servings:** 2

Ingredients:

- 2 ripe bananas
- 2 cups of fresh spinach leaves
- 1 tablespoon of flaxseeds
- 1 teaspoon of turmeric powder
- 1 cup of unsweetened almond milk
- 1 cup of ice cubes
- A small piece of fresh ginger

Directions:

1. Peel the bananas and break them into chunks.
2. Combine the banana chunks, spinach leaves, flaxseeds, turmeric powder, almond milk, ginger, and ice cubes in a blender.
3. Blend on high until the mixture is smooth and creamy. You may need to pause the blender and push down the ingredients with a spatula once or twice to ensure everything gets blended.
4. Once the smoothie is completely smooth, divide it between two glasses and serve immediately.

Calories: 160   **Protein:** 4g   **Fat:** 3g   **Carbohydrates:** 34g

4.4 Almond Flour Pancakes with a Sugar-free Berry Compote

Preparation time: 10 minutes **Cooking time:** 20 minutes **Servings:** 4

Ingredients:

For the pancakes:
- 2 Cups Almond Flour
- 4 Eggs
- 1/4 Cup Unsweetened Almond Milk
- 2 Tsp Vanilla Extract
- 1 Tbsp Baking Powder
- 2 Tbsp Erythritol or another granulated sweetener of choice
- 1/4 Tsp Salt

For the berry compote:
- 2 Cups Mixed Berries (Fresh or Frozen)
- 2 Tbsp Erythritol or another granulated sweetener of choice
- 1 Tbsp Lemon Juice
- 1/2 Tsp Vanilla Extract

Directions:

1. To make the pancakes, combine the almond flour, eggs, almond milk, vanilla extract, baking powder, erythritol, and salt in a large bowl. Mix until you have a smooth batter.
2. Heat a non-stick skillet over medium heat and lightly grease it with cooking spray or a little bit of oil. Pour about 1/4 cup of the batter onto the skillet for each pancake. Cook until bubbles form on the top and the edges look set, then flip and cook the other side. Repeat with the remaining batter.
3. While the pancakes are cooking, make the berry compote. Combine the mixed berries, erythritol, lemon juice, and vanilla extract in a saucepan. Simmer over medium heat until the berries are soft and the mixture has thickened, about 10-15 minutes.
4. Serve the pancakes with a generous spoonful of the berry compote on top.

Calories: 355   **Protein:** 15g   **Fat:** 28g   **Carbohydrates:** 14g

4.5 Greek Yogurt Parfait with Mixed Berries and Chia Seeds

Preparation time: 10 minutes

Cooking time: No cooking required

Servings: 2

Ingredients:

- 2 cups non-fat Greek yogurt
- 1 cup mixed berries (such as strawberries, blueberries, and raspberries)
- 2 tablespoons chia seeds
- 2 tablespoons honey, or to taste
- Optional toppings: granola, nuts, seeds, or additional berries

Directions:

1. Divide half of the Greek yogurt between two cups or bowls.
2. Layer half of the berries on top of the yogurt in each cup.
3. Sprinkle each cup with a tablespoon of chia seeds.
4. Drizzle each cup with a tablespoon of honey, or more to taste.
5. Repeat the layers with the remaining yogurt, berries, chia seeds, and honey.
6. Top with your choice of granola, nuts, seeds, or additional berries if desired.
7. Serve immediately, or cover and refrigerate for up to 1 day before serving.

Calories: 230   **Protein:** 18g   **Fat:** 5g   **Carbohydrates:** 31g

4.6 Chickpea Scramble with Fresh Herbs and Cherry Tomatoes

Preparation time: 10 minutes   **Cooking time:** 15 minutes   **Servings:** 4

Ingredients:

- 2 cups chickpea flour
- 2 cups water
- 1 teaspoon turmeric
- Salt and black pepper to taste
- 2 tablespoons olive oil
- 1 onion, finely chopped
- 2 garlic cloves, minced
- 1 cup cherry tomatoes, halved
- 1/2 cup chopped fresh herbs (such as parsley, cilantro, or chives)

Directions:

1. In a bowl, whisk together the chickpea flour, water, turmeric, salt, and pepper. Let sit for 5-10 minutes.
2. Heat the olive oil in a non-stick skillet over medium heat. Add the onion and garlic and sauté until soft and translucent, about 5 minutes.
3. Pour the chickpea batter into the skillet and cook, stirring frequently, until the mixture thickens and resembles scrambled eggs, about 5-7 minutes.
4. Stir in the cherry tomatoes and fresh herbs and cook for another 2-3 minutes, until the tomatoes are just starting to soften.
5. Taste and adjust the seasoning if necessary. Serve hot.

Calories: 315   **Protein:** 14g   **Fat:** 9g   **Carbohydrates:** 45g

4.7 Baked Oatmeal with Apples and Cinnamon

Preparation time: 10 minutes   **Cooking time:** 35 minutes   **Servings:** 4

Ingredients:

- 2 cups rolled oats
- 1 teaspoon baking powder
- 2 teaspoons cinnamon
- 1/4 teaspoon salt
- 1 cup almond milk (or other non-dairy milk)
- 1/4 cup maple syrup or honey
- 1 large egg
- 1 teaspoon vanilla extract
- 2 large apples, peeled, cored, and chopped
- Optional toppings: chopped nuts, seeds, or additional fresh fruit

Directions:

1. Preheat your oven to 375°F (190°C). Lightly grease a baking dish.
2. In a large bowl, combine the rolled oats, baking powder, cinnamon, and salt.
3. In another bowl, whisk together the almond milk, maple syrup or honey, egg, and vanilla extract. Pour this over the oat mixture and stir well to combine.
4. Stir in the chopped apples, then pour the mixture into your prepared baking dish.
5. Bake for 25-30 minutes, until the top is golden and the oats have set. Allow the baked oatmeal to cool for a few minutes before serving. Top with your choice of nuts, seeds, or additional fresh fruit if desired.

Calories: 295   **Protein:** 7g   **Fat:** 5g   **Carbohydrates:** 57g

4.8 Veggie Stuffed Bell Peppers with Scrambled Eggs

Preparation time: 15 minutes   **Cooking time:** 15 minutes   **Servings:** 2

Ingredients:

- 2 large bell peppers
- 4 large eggs
- 1 small onion, diced
- 1 medium tomato, diced
- 1 medium zucchini, diced
- 1 tablespoon olive oil
- Salt and pepper to taste
- Fresh herbs for garnish (like parsley or chives)

Directions:

1. Cut the tops off the bell peppers and remove the seeds and membranes. Set aside.
2. Heat the olive oil in a pan over medium heat. Add the diced onion and sauté until it becomes translucent.
3. Add the diced tomato and zucchini to the pan and continue to cook until the vegetables are softened.
4. In a separate bowl, whisk the eggs and season with salt and pepper. Pour the eggs over the cooked vegetables and stir gently, cooking until the eggs are scrambled and fully cooked.
5. Spoon the scrambled eggs and vegetables into the hollowed-out bell peppers.
6. Garnish with fresh herbs and serve warm.

Calories: 280   **Protein:** 15g   **Fat:** 16g   **Carbohydrates:** 20g

4.9 Salmon and Avocado Toast on Whole Grain Bread

Preparation time: 10 minutes   **Cooking time:** 0 minutes   **Servings:** 2

Ingredients:

- 2 slices of whole grain bread
- 1 ripe avocado
- 100g smoked salmon
- Lemon juice to taste
- Salt and pepper to taste
- Fresh dill for garnish (optional)

Directions:

1. Toast the slices of whole grain bread to your preferred level of crispiness.
2. In the meantime, slice the avocado in half, remove the pit, and scoop out the flesh. Mash it in a bowl with a fork until it's as smooth or chunky as you like it.
3. Add the lemon juice, salt, and pepper to the mashed avocado and mix well.
4. Once the toast is ready, spread half of the avocado mixture on each slice.
5. Layer the smoked salmon on top of the avocado.
6. If you like, garnish with fresh dill for an extra touch of flavor.
7. Serve immediately and enjoy this heart-healthy, satisfying breakfast!

Calories: 340   **Protein:** 19g   **Fat:** 21g   **Carbohydrates:** 23g

4.10 Protein Packed Quinoa Muffins with Blueberries

Preparation time: 20 minutes   **Cooking time:** 25 minutes   **Servings:** 12

Ingredients:

- 1 cup cooked quinoa
- 2 cups whole wheat flour
- 3/4 cup packed brown sugar
- 1 1/2 teaspoons baking powder
- 1/2 teaspoon baking soda
- 1/2 teaspoon salt
- 1 cup plain Greek yogurt
- 2 large eggs
- 1/4 cup unsweetened almond milk
- 3 tablespoons vegetable oil
- 1 teaspoon vanilla extract
- 1 cup fresh blueberries

Directions:

1. Preheat the oven to 375°F (190°C). Line a muffin tin with paper liners or lightly grease with oil.
2. In a large bowl, combine the flour, sugar, baking powder, baking soda, and salt.
3. In a separate bowl, whisk together the yogurt, eggs, almond milk, oil, and vanilla extract. Stir in the cooked quinoa.
4. Gradually add the wet ingredients to the dry ingredients, mixing just until combined. Be careful not to overmix.
5. Gently fold in the blueberries.
6. Divide the batter evenly among the muffin cups, filling each about 3/4 full.
7. Bake for 20-25 minutes, or until a toothpick inserted into the center of a muffin comes out clean.
8. Allow the muffins to cool in the pan for 5 minutes, then transfer them to a wire rack to cool completely.

Calories: 210   **Protein:** 6g   **Fat:** 5g   **Carbohydrates:** 35g

4.11 Huevos Rancheros with Whole Grain Tortilla and Fresh Salsa

Preparation time: 15 minutes   **Cooking time:** 20 minutes   **Servings:** 4

Ingredients:

For the Fresh Salsa:

- 2 ripe tomatoes, diced
- 1 small red onion, finely chopped
- 1 jalapeno, seeds removed and finely chopped
- 1/4 cup chopped fresh cilantro
- Juice of 1 lime
- Salt, to taste

For the Huevos Rancheros:

- 4 whole grain tortillas
- 4 large eggs
- 1 can (15 oz) black beans, rinsed and drained
- 1 avocado, sliced
- 1/4 cup crumbled queso fresco or feta cheese
- Olive oil, for cooking
- Salt and pepper, to taste

Directions:

1. First, prepare the salsa. In a bowl, combine the tomatoes, onion, jalapeno, cilantro, and lime juice. Season with salt and mix well. Set aside to allow the flavors to meld together.
2. Heat a small amount of olive oil in a large skillet over medium heat. Add the eggs and cook until the whites are set but the yolks are still runny, about 3-4 minutes. Season with salt and pepper.
3. While the eggs are cooking, warm the tortillas in a dry skillet over medium heat until they are soft and pliable.
4. To assemble, spread a layer of black beans on each tortilla. Top with a fried egg, a generous spoonful of salsa, a few slices of avocado, and a sprinkle of cheese.
5. Serve immediately, with additional salsa on the side if desired.

Calories: 325   **Protein:** 15g   **Fat:** 15g   **Carbohydrates:** 35g

4.12 Oatmeal Smoothie with Banana, Blueberries, and Almond Milk

Preparation time: 5 minutes   **Cooking time:** 0 minutes   **Servings:** 1

Ingredients:

- 1 ripe banana
- 1 cup of fresh or frozen blueberries
- 1/4 cup of raw oats
- 1 cup of unsweetened almond milk
- A handful of ice cubes (optional)

Directions:

1. Place the banana, blueberries, oats, and almond milk into a blender.
2. Blend on high until all the ingredients are well combined and the smoothie is creamy. If you prefer a colder smoothie, add the ice cubes and blend again until smooth.
3. Pour the smoothie into a glass or smoothie bottle if you're on the go.
4. Enjoy this fiber-rich, antioxidant-packed breakfast smoothie immediately for the best flavor and texture.

Calories: 290   **Protein:** 7g   **Fat:** 5g   **Carbohydrates:** 60g

4.13 Vegetable Frittata with Spinach, Bell Peppers, and Zucchini

Preparation time: 15 minutes   **Cooking   time: 20   Servings:** 4

minutes

Ingredients:

- 6 Large Eggs
- 1/4 Cup Almond Milk
- 1 Cup Fresh Spinach, Chopped
- 1 Bell Pepper, Diced
- 1 Small Zucchini, Sliced
- 2 Cloves Garlic, Minced
- 1 Small Onion, Diced
- 1 Tbsp Olive Oil
- Salt and Pepper to Taste

Directions:

1. Preheat your oven to 375 degrees F (190 degrees C).
2. In a large bowl, beat together the eggs and almond milk. Season with a little salt and pepper. Set aside.
3. In an oven-safe skillet, heat the olive oil over medium heat. Add the onion and garlic, and cook until they become translucent.
4. Add the bell pepper and zucchini to the skillet, and sauté until they're soft.
5. Add the spinach to the skillet and cook until wilted.
6. Pour the egg mixture over the vegetables in the skillet, stirring gently to distribute the vegetables evenly.
7. Transfer the skillet to the preheated oven and bake for about 15 minutes, or until the frittata is set and slightly golden on top.
8. Let the frittata cool for a few minutes before slicing and serving.

Calories: 180   **Protein:** 12g   **Fat:** 11g   **Carbohydrates:** 7g

4.14 Vegetable and Egg Muffins with Kale, Onion, and Bell Pepper

Preparation time: 15 minutes   **Cooking time:** 25 minutes   **Servings:** 6 (two muffins per serving)

Ingredients:

- 12 large eggs
- 1 cup kale, finely chopped
- 1/2 cup bell pepper, finely diced
- 1/2 cup onion, finely diced
- Salt and pepper to taste
- 1/2 teaspoon garlic powder
- Olive oil or cooking spray for the muffin pan

Directions:

1. Preheat your oven to 350°F (175°C). Lightly grease a 12-cup muffin pan with olive oil or cooking spray.
2. In a large bowl, beat the eggs. Add the kale, bell pepper, onion, salt, pepper, and garlic powder. Stir until well combined.
3. Pour the egg and vegetable mixture evenly into the muffin cups.
4. Bake in the preheated oven for 20-25 minutes, or until the tops are firm to the touch and eggs are cooked.
5. Allow the muffins to cool for a few minutes before removing from the muffin pan. Serve warm.

Calories: 215   **Protein:** 18g   **Fat:** 14g   **Carbohydrates:** 3g

4.15 Buckwheat Pancakes with Fresh Fruit and Sugar-free Maple Syrup

Preparation time: 10 minutes   **Cooking time:** 15 minutes   **Servings:** 4 (two pancakes per serving)

Ingredients:

- 1 cup buckwheat flour
- 1 cup almond milk
- 1 tablespoon honey or other natural sweetener
- 1 egg
- 1/2 teaspoon baking powder
- Pinch of salt
- 1 teaspoon vanilla extract
- Coconut oil or cooking spray for the pan
- Fresh fruit for topping (berries, sliced bananas, etc.)
- Sugar-free maple syrup for serving

Directions:

1. In a large bowl, mix together the buckwheat flour, baking powder, and salt.
2. In another bowl, whisk together the almond milk, egg, honey, and vanilla extract.
3. Gradually add the wet ingredients to the dry ingredients, stirring until the batter is smooth.
4. Heat a non-stick skillet over medium heat and lightly grease with coconut oil or cooking spray.
5. Pour 1/4 cup of batter for each pancake onto the skillet. Cook until bubbles form on the surface, then flip and cook until browned on the other side.
6. Serve the pancakes topped with fresh fruit and a drizzle of sugar-free maple syrup.

Calories: 170   **Protein:** 6g   **Fat:** 3g   **Carbohydrates:** 32g

5 Lunch Recipes

5.1 Lemon Baked Salmon with Dill and Asparagus

Preparation time: 10 minutes   **Cooking time:** 20 minutes   **Servings:** 4

Ingredients:

- 4 salmon fillets (about 6 ounces each)
- 1 bunch asparagus, trimmed
- 3 tablespoons olive oil
- 1 lemon, zested and juiced
- 2 tablespoons fresh dill, chopped
- Salt and pepper to taste

Directions:

1. Preheat the oven to 400°F (200°C). Line a large baking sheet with parchment paper.
2. Arrange the salmon fillets and asparagus on the prepared baking sheet. Drizzle with olive oil and lemon juice, then sprinkle with lemon zest, dill, salt, and pepper.
3. Bake for about 15-20 minutes, or until the salmon is cooked to your desired doneness and the asparagus is tender.
4. Serve the salmon and asparagus hot, garnished with additional fresh dill if desired.

Calories: 350   **Protein:** 35g   **Fat:** 20g   **Carbohydrates:** 7g

5.2 Grilled Chicken Breast with Quinoa and Steamed Broccoli

Preparation time: 10 minutes   **Cooking time:** 25 minutes   **Servings:** 4

Ingredients:

- 4 chicken breasts (about 1.5 pounds)
- 1 cup quinoa, uncooked
- 1 large head of broccoli, cut into florets
- 2 tablespoons of olive oil
- Salt and pepper to taste
- 1 lemon, zested and juiced
- 2 cloves of garlic, minced

Directions:

1. Rinse the quinoa under cold water and drain. In a medium-sized saucepan, cook quinoa according to package instructions.
2. While the quinoa is cooking, season chicken breasts with salt, pepper, half of the lemon zest, and minced garlic.
3. Heat a grill pan over medium heat and add one tablespoon of olive oil. Once the oil is hot, add the chicken breasts. Cook for about 6-7 minutes on each side or until the chicken is no longer pink in the middle.
4. Meanwhile, steam the broccoli until it's tender yet crisp - this should take about 5 minutes.
5. Once everything is ready, divide the quinoa, grilled chicken, and steamed broccoli evenly among four plates.
6. Drizzle each plate with the remaining olive oil, lemon juice, and sprinkle with the remaining lemon zest. Add additional salt and pepper to taste if needed.

Calories: 410   **Protein:** 50g   **Fat:** 10g   **Carbohydrates:** 25g

5.3 Lentil Soup with Carrots, Celery, and Onions

Preparation time: 15 minutes   **Cooking time:** 1 hour   **Servings:** 6

Ingredients:

- 2 cups dried lentils
- 1 tablespoon olive oil
- 1 large onion, diced
- 2 carrots, diced
- 2 stalks celery, diced
- 4 cloves garlic, minced
- 6 cups vegetable broth
- 1 teaspoon dried thyme
- Salt and pepper to taste
- Fresh parsley, chopped (for garnish)

Directions:

1. Rinse the lentils under cold water and set aside.
2. In a large pot, heat the olive oil over medium heat. Add the onion, carrots, and celery, and cook until the vegetables are tender, about 5-7 minutes. Add the garlic and cook for another minute.
3. Add the lentils, vegetable broth, and thyme to the pot. Bring to a boil, then reduce heat and simmer, covered, for about 50-60 minutes, or until lentils are soft.
4. Season the soup with salt and pepper to taste. You can puree part of the soup with an immersion blender for a creamier texture if desired.
5. Ladle the soup into bowls and garnish with fresh parsley before serving.

Calories: 300   **Protein:** 18g   **Fat:** 3g   **Carbohydrates:** 50g

5.4 Veggie Wrap with Whole Grain Tortilla and Hummus

Preparation time: 10 minutes   **Cooking time:** 0 minutes   **Servings:** 2

Ingredients:

- 2 whole grain tortillas
- 4 tablespoons hummus
- 1 carrot, grated
- 1/2 cucumber, thinly sliced
- 1 bell pepper, thinly sliced
- 1/2 cup baby spinach leaves
- Salt and pepper to taste

Directions:

1. Lay out the whole grain tortillas on a flat surface.
2. Spread 2 tablespoons of hummus evenly onto each tortilla.
3. In the center of each tortilla, place half of the grated carrot, cucumber slices, bell pepper slices, and baby spinach leaves.
4. Season the vegetables with salt and pepper to taste.
5. Roll up the tortillas tightly, tucking in the ends as you go. Cut each wrap in half before serving.

Calories: 200   **Protein:** 8g   **Fat:** 7g   **Carbohydrates:** 32g

5.5 Shrimp Stir Fry with Bell Peppers, Zucchini, and Brown Rice

Preparation time: 15 minutes   **Cooking time:** 20 minutes   **Servings:** 4

Ingredients:

- 1 cup brown rice
- 2 cups water
- 1 lb shrimp, peeled and deveined
- 1 bell pepper, sliced
- 1 zucchini, sliced

- 1 tablespoon olive oil
- 2 cloves garlic, minced
- 1 tablespoon low-sodium soy sauce
- 1 teaspoon sesame oil
- Salt and pepper to taste

Directions:

1. Rinse the brown rice under cold water until the water runs clear. Add the rice and water to a saucepan and bring to a boil. Reduce heat to low, cover, and let simmer for about 45 minutes, or until the rice is cooked and the water is absorbed. Set aside.
2. While the rice is cooking, heat the olive oil in a large pan over medium heat. Add the garlic and cook for a minute until fragrant.
3. Add the bell pepper and zucchini to the pan and cook for 5 minutes, or until the vegetables are tender.
4. Add the shrimp to the pan and cook for 2-3 minutes on each side, or until the shrimp are pink and cooked through.
5. Stir in the soy sauce and sesame oil. Season with salt and pepper to taste.
6. Serve the shrimp and vegetable stir fry over the cooked brown rice.

Calories: 330   **Protein:** 26g   **Fat:** 6g   **Carbohydrates:** 40g

5.6 Baked Sweet Potato with Black Beans and Salsa

Preparation time: 10 minutes   **Cooking time:** 45 minutes   **Servings:** 4

Ingredients:

- 4 medium sweet potatoes
- 1 can (15 oz) black beans, rinsed and drained
- 1 cup salsa
- 1 avocado, diced

- 1 lime, cut into wedges
- Fresh cilantro, chopped (optional)
- Salt and pepper to taste

Directions:

1. Preheat your oven to 400°F (200°C). Prick the sweet potatoes all over with a fork and place them on a baking sheet.
2. Bake the sweet potatoes in the preheated oven for 40-50 minutes, or until tender when pierced with a fork.
3. While the sweet potatoes are baking, heat the black beans in a small saucepan over medium heat.
4. Slice open the baked sweet potatoes and lightly fluff the insides with a fork.
5. Spoon the warm black beans onto each sweet potato. Top with salsa and diced avocado.
6. Garnish with fresh cilantro if desired and serve with a lime wedge.

Calories: 360   **Protein:** 12g   **Fat:** 8g   **Carbohydrates:** 65g

5.7 Grilled Turkey Burger with Avocado and Sweet Potato Fries

Preparation time: 20 minutes   **Cooking time:** 30 minutes   **Servings:** 4

Ingredients:

For the Turkey Burger:

- 1 lb ground turkey
- 1 medium-sized avocado, sliced

For the Sweet Potato Fries:

- 2 large sweet potatoes
- 1 tbsp olive oil

- 4 whole grain hamburger buns
- Lettuce, tomato, and onion for garnish

- Salt and pepper to taste

Directions:

1. Preheat your grill and your oven to 400°F (200°C).
2. Peel the sweet potatoes and cut them into fries. Toss the sweet potato fries with olive oil, salt, and pepper. Spread them out on a baking sheet and bake for 20-30 minutes, flipping once, until crispy.
3. While the sweet potatoes are baking, form the ground turkey into four patties. Season each patty with salt and pepper.
4. Grill the turkey burgers for 5-6 minutes per side, or until the internal temperature reaches 165°F (74°C).
5. Assemble the turkey burgers on the whole grain buns with lettuce, tomato, onion, and slices of avocado. Serve with the sweet potato fries on the side.

Calories: 500   **Protein:** 30g   **Fat:** 23g   **Carbohydrates:** 45g

5.8 Baked Cod with Lemon, Capers, and Roasted Brussels Sprouts

Preparation time: 15 minutes   **Cooking time:** 25 minutes   **Servings:** 4

Ingredients:

- 4 cod fillets
- 1 lemon, thinly sliced
- 2 tbsp capers, drained
- Salt and pepper to taste

- 2 tbsp olive oil
- 1 lb Brussels sprouts, halved
- 2 garlic cloves, minced

Directions:

1. Preheat your oven to 400°F (200°C).
2. In a large bowl, toss the Brussels sprouts with 1 tbsp of olive oil, minced garlic, salt, and pepper.
3. Spread the Brussels sprouts out on a baking sheet and roast for 20-25 minutes, until crispy and tender.
4. While the Brussels sprouts are roasting, season the cod fillets with salt and pepper. Drizzle with remaining olive oil, and top each fillet with a few slices of lemon and a sprinkling of capers.
5. Bake the cod in a baking dish for about 15 minutes, or until the fish is opaque and flakes easily with a fork.
6. Serve the baked cod with the roasted Brussels sprouts on the side.

Calories: 280   **Protein:** 30g   **Fat:** 10g   **Carbohydrates:** 15g

5.9 Whole Grain Pasta with Tomato Sauce and Steamed Vegetables

Preparation time: 10 minutes **Cooking time:** 20 minutes **Servings:** 4

Ingredients:

- 8 ounces whole grain spaghetti
- 1 tablespoon olive oil
- 1 onion, chopped
- 2 cloves garlic, minced
- 1 can (14.5 ounces) diced tomatoes

- 1/2 teaspoon dried basil
- 1/2 teaspoon dried oregano
- Salt and pepper to taste
- 4 cups of mixed vegetables (broccoli, cauliflower, carrots, bell peppers)

Directions:

1. Cook the pasta according to the package instructions until al dente. Drain and set aside.
2. While the pasta is cooking, heat the olive oil in a large pan over medium heat. Add the chopped onion and minced garlic, and sauté until the onion is translucent and the garlic is fragrant.
3. Add the diced tomatoes (with juice), basil, oregano, and salt and pepper to the pan. Bring the mixture to a simmer and let it cook for about 10 minutes, until the sauce has thickened.
4. Meanwhile, steam your mixed vegetables until they are just tender, about 5-7 minutes.
5. Once the vegetables are cooked and the sauce has thickened, add the cooked pasta to the pan with the sauce and stir well to combine.
6. Divide the pasta and sauce among 4 plates, top each with an equal amount of the steamed vegetables, and serve immediately.

Calories: 350   **Protein:** 13g   **Fat:** 7g   **Carbohydrates:** 60g

5.10 Quinoa Salad with Avocado, Black Beans, and Corn

Preparation time: 15 minutes **Cooking time:** 20 minutes **Servings:** 4

Ingredients:

- 1 cup quinoa
- 2 cups water
- 1 can black beans, drained and rinsed
- 1 cup corn kernels (fresh or frozen)
- 2 ripe avocados, diced
- 1 red bell pepper, diced

- 1/2 red onion, finely chopped
- 1/4 cup chopped fresh cilantro
- Juice of 1 lime
- 2 tablespoons olive oil
- Salt and pepper to taste

Directions:

1. Rinse the quinoa under cold water until the water runs clear.
2. In a medium saucepan, bring the water to a boil. Add the quinoa, reduce heat to low, cover, and simmer until quinoa is tender and the water has been absorbed, about 15 minutes. Allow to cool.
3. In a large bowl, combine cooled quinoa, black beans, corn, avocados, bell pepper, and onion.
4. In a small bowl, whisk together the lime juice, olive oil, and a pinch of salt and pepper to create a dressing.
5. Pour the dressing over the quinoa mixture and toss gently to combine. Sprinkle with cilantro.
6. This salad can be served immediately, or refrigerated for a couple of hours to allow the flavors to meld together.

Calories: 380   **Protein:** 10g   **Fat:** 16g   **Carbohydrates:** 50g

5.11 Avocado Tuna Salad with Whole Grain Crackers

Preparation time: 10 minutes   **Cooking time:** 0 minutes   **Servings:** 4

Ingredients:

- 2 cans (5 oz each) tuna in water, drained
- 1 ripe avocado, pitted and peeled
- 1 tablespoon lemon juice
- 1/4 cup red onion, finely chopped
- 1/2 cup celery, finely chopped
- Salt and pepper to taste
- 16 whole grain crackers

Directions:

1. In a medium bowl, mash the avocado with the lemon juice until relatively smooth.
2. Add the drained tuna to the bowl, breaking it up with a fork and mixing it with the mashed avocado.
3. Add the chopped red onion and celery to the bowl. Stir everything together until it's well combined.
4. Season the mixture with salt and pepper to taste.
5. Serve the avocado tuna salad immediately, or refrigerate it for later use. Serve with whole grain crackers on the side.

Calories: 220   **Protein:** 19g   **Fat:** 10g   **Carbohydrates:** 18g

5.12 Vegetable Curry with Chickpeas and Basmati Rice

Preparation time: 20 minutes   **Cooking time:** 30 minutes   **Servings:** 4

Ingredients:

- 1 cup Basmati rice
- 2 cups water
- 1 tablespoon olive oil
- 1 onion, chopped
- 2 cloves garlic, minced
- 1 tablespoon curry powder
- 1 teaspoon turmeric
- 1 can chickpeas, drained and rinsed
- 1 cup diced tomatoes (fresh or canned)
- 1 cup broccoli florets
- 1 cup diced bell peppers
- 1 cup chopped carrots
- 1 can coconut milk
- Salt and pepper to taste
- Fresh cilantro, chopped (for garnish)

Directions:

1. In a medium saucepan, bring water to a boil. Add the Basmati rice, reduce the heat to low, cover, and simmer for 15-20 minutes until the rice is cooked and the water has been absorbed.
2. While the rice is cooking, heat olive oil in a large pan over medium heat. Add the onion and garlic, sautéing until the onion becomes translucent.
3. Add the curry powder and turmeric, stirring to coat the onion and garlic.
4. Add the chickpeas, diced tomatoes, broccoli, bell peppers, and carrots to the pan. Cook for 5-10 minutes until the vegetables are tender.
5. Stir in the coconut milk, bringing the mixture to a simmer. Season with salt and pepper to taste.
6. Let the curry simmer for about 10 minutes until it thickens slightly.
7. Serve the vegetable curry over the cooked Basmati rice. Garnish with fresh cilantro.

Calories: 520   **Protein:** 13g   **Fat:** 19g   **Carbohydrates:** 77g

5.13 Stuffed Bell Peppers with Ground Turkey and Brown Rice

Preparation time: 25 minutes   **Cooking time:** 35 minutes   **Servings:** 4

Ingredients:

- 4 bell peppers, any color
- 1 cup cooked brown rice
- 1 lb lean ground turkey
- 1 small onion, diced
- 2 cloves garlic, minced
- 1 can diced tomatoes, drained
- 1/2 cup shredded low-fat cheese
- 1 teaspoon olive oil
- Salt and pepper to taste
- Fresh parsley, chopped (for garnish)

Directions:

1. Preheat the oven to 375°F (190°C).
2. Cut the tops off the bell peppers and remove the seeds and membranes. Set aside.
3. Heat the olive oil in a large skillet over medium heat. Add the onion and garlic, sautéing until the onion is translucent.
4. Add the ground turkey to the skillet. Cook until it's no longer pink, breaking it up into small pieces as it cooks.
5. Add the cooked brown rice and diced tomatoes to the skillet, stirring to combine. Season with salt and pepper to taste.
6. Spoon the turkey and rice mixture into the hollowed-out bell peppers. Place the peppers in a baking dish.
7. Top each pepper with a sprinkle of shredded cheese.
8. Bake for 30-35 minutes until the peppers are tender and the cheese is melted and slightly browned.
9. Garnish with fresh parsley before serving.

Calories: 360   **Protein:** 30g   **Fat:** 13g   **Carbohydrates:** 28g

5.14 Steamed Fish with Ginger, Garlic, and Mixed Vegetables

Preparation time: 15 minutes   **Cooking time:** 20 minutes   **Servings:** 4

Ingredients:

- 4 white fish fillets (such as cod or halibut)
- 2 inches of fresh ginger, peeled and thinly sliced
- 4 cloves of garlic, minced
- 2 cups of mixed vegetables (like bell peppers, zucchini, and carrots), thinly sliced
- Salt and pepper to taste
- 2 tablespoons of soy sauce
- 1 tablespoon of sesame oil
- Green onions and fresh cilantro for garnish

Directions:

1. Rinse the fish fillets and pat dry. Season with salt and pepper on both sides.
2. Arrange a bed of mixed vegetables on the bottom of the steaming basket.
3. Place the fish fillets on top of the vegetables. Sprinkle the ginger and garlic evenly over the fish.
4. Set up your steamer, ensuring the water level doesn't touch the bottom of the steamer basket. Cover and steam over medium-high heat for about 10-12 minutes, or until the fish is cooked through and flaky.
5. Meanwhile, mix together the soy sauce and sesame oil in a small bowl.
6. Once the fish is cooked, carefully remove the steaming basket from the heat. Drizzle the soy sauce mixture over the fish and vegetables.
7. Garnish with green onions and fresh cilantro before serving.

Calories: 220   **Protein:** 28g   **Fat:** 8g   **Carbohydrates:** 8g

5.15 Greek Salad with Grilled Chicken Breast

Preparation time: 20 minutes   **Cooking time:** 20 minutes   **Servings:** 4

Ingredients:

- 4 boneless, skinless chicken breasts
- 1 tablespoon olive oil
- Salt and pepper to taste
- 1 head romaine lettuce, chopped
- 2 tomatoes, diced
- 1 cucumber, sliced
- 1 red onion, thinly sliced
- 1/2 cup Kalamata olives
- 1/2 cup feta cheese, crumbled
- For the dressing: 1/4 cup olive oil, 2 tablespoons red wine vinegar, 1 teaspoon dried oregano, Salt and pepper to taste

Directions:

1. Preheat your grill or grill pan over medium heat.
2. Rub the chicken breasts with olive oil and season with salt and pepper.
3. Grill the chicken for 6-7 minutes on each side, or until it's cooked through and no longer pink in the middle. Set aside to cool, then slice into strips.
4. While the chicken is cooling, prepare your salad. In a large bowl, combine the lettuce, tomatoes, cucumber, red onion, olives, and feta cheese.
5. For the dressing, whisk together the olive oil, red wine vinegar, dried oregano, salt, and pepper. Adjust the seasoning to your liking.
6. Drizzle the dressing over the salad and toss to combine.
7. Top the salad with the grilled chicken strips before serving.

Calories: 400   **Protein:** 35g   **Fat:** 25g   **Carbohydrates:** 10g

6 Dinner Recipes

6.1 Chicken and Vegetable Stir Fry with Brown Rice

Preparation time: 15 minutes   **Cooking time:** 20 minutes   **Servings:** 4

Ingredients:

- 2 boneless, skinless chicken breasts, cut into strips
- 2 cups of brown rice, cooked
- 2 cups of broccoli florets
- 1 red bell pepper, sliced
- 1 yellow bell pepper, sliced
- 1 medium onion, sliced
- 2 cloves of garlic, minced
- 2 tablespoons of olive oil
- 1/4 cup of low sodium soy sauce (or tamari for gluten-free)
- 1 teaspoon of ginger, grated
- Salt and pepper to taste
- Optional garnish: sesame seeds, sliced green onions

Directions:

1. In a large pan or wok, heat one tablespoon of olive oil over medium heat. Add the chicken strips and season with salt and pepper. Cook until no longer pink in the middle, about 5-7 minutes. Remove from the pan and set aside.
2. In the same pan, add another tablespoon of olive oil. Add in the broccoli, bell peppers, and onion. Stir fry for about 5 minutes, until the vegetables are tender but still have a bit of crunch.
3. Add the garlic and ginger to the pan, and cook for another minute until fragrant.
4. Return the chicken to the pan. Pour the soy sauce over everything and toss well to combine, ensuring the chicken and vegetables are well coated.
5. Serve the stir fry over the cooked brown rice. Garnish with sesame seeds and sliced green onions if desired.

Calories: 410   **Protein:** 28g   **Fat:** 10g   **Carbohydrates:** 52g

6.2 Baked Lemon Herb Salmon with Quinoa and Asparagus

Preparation time: 10 minutes   **Cooking time:** 20 minutes   **Servings:** 4

Ingredients:

- 4 salmon fillets
- 2 cups of quinoa, cooked
- 1 pound of asparagus, ends trimmed
- 2 tablespoons of olive oil
- 1 lemon, sliced plus juice of half a lemon
- 4 cloves of garlic, minced
- 2 tablespoons of fresh dill, chopped
- Salt and pepper to taste

Directions:

1. Preheat your oven to 400 degrees F (200 degrees C) and line a baking sheet with foil or parchment paper.
2. Lay the salmon fillets on the lined baking sheet and surround with asparagus spears.
3. Drizzle the olive oil and lemon juice over the salmon and asparagus. Sprinkle with the minced garlic, chopped dill, salt, and pepper. Lay the lemon slices on top of the salmon fillets.
4. Bake in the preheated oven for about 15-20 minutes, or until the salmon is cooked through and the asparagus is tender.
5. Serve the salmon and asparagus over a bed of cooked quinoa. You can drizzle the cooking juices on top for extra flavor.

Calories: 450   **Protein:** 35g   **Fat:** 16g   **Carbohydrates:** 42g

6.3 Grilled Shrimp Tacos with Avocado Salsa

Preparation time: 15 minutes   **Cooking time:** 10 minutes   **Servings:** 4

Ingredients:

- 1 lb large shrimp, peeled and deveined
- 8 small whole grain tortillas
- 1 ripe avocado, diced
- 1/2 cup diced tomatoes
- 1/4 cup chopped red onion
- 1 jalapeño, seeds removed and finely diced
- 1/4 cup chopped fresh cilantro
- Juice of 1 lime
- Salt and pepper to taste
- 1 tablespoon olive oil
- 1/2 teaspoon chili powder
- 1/2 teaspoon ground cumin
- 1/4 teaspoon garlic powder

Directions:

1. Preheat grill to medium-high heat.
2. In a large bowl, mix together the olive oil, chili powder, cumin, garlic powder, and salt and pepper. Add the shrimp and toss until they are evenly coated.
3. Thread the shrimp onto skewers and grill for 2-3 minutes per side, until they are opaque and cooked through.
4. While the shrimp are grilling, make the avocado salsa. In a medium bowl, combine the diced avocado, tomatoes, red onion, jalapeño, cilantro, and lime juice. Season with salt and pepper and toss until well combined.
5. Warm the tortillas on the grill for a few seconds on each side.
6. To assemble the tacos, divide the grilled shrimp evenly among the tortillas and top with the avocado salsa.

Calories: 370   **Protein:** 30g   **Fat:** 15g   **Carbohydrates:** 30g

6.4 Vegan Buddha Bowl with Roasted Sweet Potatoes and Quinoa

Preparation time: 15 minutes   **Cooking time:** 30 minutes   **Servings:** 4

Ingredients:

- 2 large sweet potatoes, peeled and cut into cubes
- 1 cup uncooked quinoa
- 2 cups water
- 2 cups fresh spinach
- 1 can chickpeas, drained and rinsed

- 2 avocados, sliced
- 1/4 cup olive oil
- Salt and pepper to taste
- 1 teaspoon paprika
- 1/2 teaspoon garlic powder

For the Dressing:

- 2 tablespoons tahini
- 1 tablespoon maple syrup
- Juice of 1 lemon

- 2-3 tablespoons water
- Salt to taste

Directions:

1. Preheat your oven to 400 degrees F. Toss the sweet potatoes with 2 tablespoons of olive oil, paprika, garlic powder, salt, and pepper. Spread them out on a baking sheet and roast for 25-30 minutes, until they are tender and slightly browned.
2. While the sweet potatoes are roasting, cook the quinoa. Combine the quinoa and water in a saucepan, bring to a boil, then reduce heat and simmer for 15 minutes until all water is absorbed.

3. For the dressing, mix the tahini, maple syrup, and lemon juice in a bowl. Add water one tablespoon at a time until you reach your desired consistency. Season with salt.
4. To assemble the bowls, divide the quinoa evenly among four bowls. Top each with a portion of the roasted sweet potatoes, fresh spinach, chickpeas, and sliced avocado. Drizzle with the tahini dressing and serve.

Calories: 570   **Protein:** 15g   **Fat:** 25g   **Carbohydrates:** 70g

6.5 Zucchini Noodles with Tomato and Basil Sauce

Preparation time: 15 minutes   **Cooking time:** 15 minutes   **Servings:** 4

Ingredients:

- 4 large zucchinis
- 2 tablespoons olive oil
- 2 cloves garlic, minced
- 1 onion, chopped

- 1 can (28 ounces) crushed tomatoes
- 1/4 cup fresh basil leaves, torn
- Salt and pepper to taste

Directions:

1. Spiralize the zucchinis to create noodles, or cut into thin strips if you don't have a spiralizer. Set aside.
2. In a large skillet, heat the olive oil over medium heat. Add the garlic and onion and sauté until they are soft and fragrant.
3. Add the crushed tomatoes to the skillet and bring the sauce to a simmer.
4. Let the sauce simmer for about 10 minutes to allow the flavors to blend together.

5. While the sauce is simmering, heat another skillet over medium heat. Add the zucchini noodles and cook for 2-3 minutes until they are just tender. Be careful not to overcook them, or they will become mushy.
6. Season the tomato sauce with salt and pepper to taste, and stir in the torn basil leaves.
7. Serve the zucchini noodles topped with the tomato and basil sauce.

Calories: 180   **Protein:** 5g   **Fat:** 10g   **Carbohydrates:** 20g

6.6 Beef and Broccoli Stir Fry with Jasmine Rice

Preparation time: 15 minutes   **Cooking time:** 20 minutes   **Servings:** 4

Ingredients:

- 1 lb lean beef steak, cut into thin strips
- 2 cups broccoli florets
- 1 cup jasmine rice

For the Sauce:
- 1/2 cup low sodium soy sauce
- 1 tablespoon cornstarch
- 1 tablespoon brown sugar

- 2 tablespoons vegetable oil
- 1 onion, sliced
- 2 cloves garlic, minced

- 1 teaspoon ginger, minced
- 1/2 cup beef broth

Directions:

1. Cook the jasmine rice according to the package instructions and set aside.
2. In a large wok or skillet, heat the oil over medium-high heat. Add the beef and stir fry until it is fully cooked. Remove the beef from the pan and set aside.
3. In the same pan, add the onion and garlic, and cook until the onion is translucent.
4. Add the broccoli florets to the pan and cook for a few minutes until they are tender.
5. In a small bowl, whisk together the soy sauce, cornstarch, brown sugar, ginger, and beef broth. Pour the sauce over the cooked vegetables in the pan and bring the mixture to a simmer.
6. Return the beef to the pan and stir everything together. Cook for a few more minutes until the sauce has thickened.
7. Serve the beef and broccoli over the cooked jasmine rice.

Calories: 450   **Protein:** 30g   **Fat:** 15g   **Carbohydrates:** 48g

6.7 Baked Cod with Lemon and Dill, served with Steamed Green Beans

Preparation time: 10 minutes   **Cooking time:** 20 minutes   **Servings:** 4

Ingredients:

- 4 cod fillets
- 2 lemons, sliced
- 4 tablespoons fresh dill, chopped
- Salt and pepper to taste

- 2 tablespoons olive oil
- 1 pound green beans, trimmed
- Lemon wedges for serving

Directions:

1. Preheat your oven to 400 degrees F (200 degrees C). Line a baking sheet with parchment paper.
2. Arrange the cod fillets on the prepared baking sheet. Season each fillet with salt and pepper.
3. Drizzle the olive oil over the cod fillets. Arrange the lemon slices on top of each fillet, then sprinkle with the chopped dill.
4. Bake the cod in the preheated oven for about 15-20 minutes, or until the fish is opaque and flakes easily with a fork.
5. While the fish is baking, steam the green beans until they are tender but still crisp. Season with salt and pepper to taste.
6. Serve the baked cod hot, with the steamed green beans on the side. Add a lemon wedge for squeezing over the fish.

Calories: 230   **Protein:** 30g   **Fat:** 8g   **Carbohydrates:** 10g

6.8 Turkey Meatball and Vegetable Soup with Whole Grain Bread

Preparation time: 20 minutes   **Cooking time:** 30 minutes   **Servings:** 6

Ingredients:

- Whole grain bread for serving

For the Meatballs:

- 1 pound ground turkey
- 1/4 cup whole grain breadcrumbs
- 1/4 cup Parmesan cheese, grated
- 1 egg
- 2 tablespoons fresh parsley, chopped
- Salt and pepper to taste

For the soup:

- 2 tablespoons olive oil
- 1 onion, diced
- 2 carrots, diced
- 2 stalks celery, diced
- 4 cloves garlic, minced
- 1 can (28 ounces) diced tomatoes
- 6 cups chicken broth
- 1 teaspoon dried basil
- Salt and pepper to taste
- 2 cups fresh spinach leaves

Directions:

1. Start by making the meatballs. In a large bowl, combine the ground turkey, breadcrumbs, Parmesan cheese, egg, parsley, salt, and pepper. Mix well until all the ingredients are evenly distributed.
2. Form the mixture into 1-inch meatballs and set them aside.
3. In a large pot, heat the olive oil over medium heat. Add the onion, carrots, celery, and garlic, and sauté until the vegetables are soft.
4. Add the diced tomatoes, chicken broth, and dried basil to the pot. Season with salt and pepper to taste.
5. Gently add the meatballs to the pot. Let the soup simmer for about 20 minutes, until the meatballs are cooked through.
6. Just before serving, stir in the fresh spinach leaves and let them wilt in the hot soup.
7. Serve the soup hot, with whole grain bread on the side.

Calories: 330   **Protein:** 25g   **Fat:** 12g   **Carbohydrates:** 30g

6.9 One-Pan Lemon Garlic Shrimp and Asparagus

Preparation time: 15 minutes   **Cooking time:** 20 minutes   **Servings:** 4

Ingredients:

- 1 lb. large shrimp, peeled and deveined
- 1 lb. asparagus, ends trimmed
- 3 tablespoons olive oil
- 4 garlic cloves, minced
- Zest and juice of 1 lemon
- Salt and pepper to taste
- Red chili flakes (optional)
- Fresh parsley, chopped (for garnish)

Directions:

1. Preheat your oven to 400°F (200°C) and line a large baking sheet with parchment paper.
2. In a large mixing bowl, combine the shrimp, asparagus, olive oil, garlic, lemon zest, and lemon juice. Toss to coat, then season with salt, pepper, and chili flakes if using.
3. Spread the shrimp and asparagus out in a single layer on the prepared baking sheet.
4. Bake for 12-15 minutes, or until the shrimp are pink and cooked through, and the asparagus is tender.
5. Garnish with freshly chopped parsley before serving. This dish pairs wonderfully with whole grain bread or quinoa for a complete meal.

Calories: 230   **Protein:** 24g   **Fat:** 12g   **Carbohydrates:** 7g

6.10 Sweet Potato and Black Bean Chili with Cornbread

Preparation time: 15 minutes   **Cooking time:** 45 minutes   **Servings:** 6

Ingredients:

For the Chili:

- 2 tablespoons olive oil
- 1 medium onion, diced
- 2 cloves garlic, minced
- 1 large sweet potato, peeled and diced
- 2 tablespoons chili powder
- 1 teaspoon ground cumin
- 1/4 teaspoon cayenne pepper (optional)
- 2 cans (15 oz each) black beans, rinsed and drained
- 1 can (14.5 oz) diced tomatoes
- 4 cups vegetable broth
- Salt and pepper to taste

For the Cornbread:

- 1 cup cornmeal
- 1 cup all-purpose flour
- 1/4 cup sugar
- 1 tablespoon baking powder
- 1/2 teaspoon salt
- 1 cup milk
- 1/3 cup vegetable oil
- 1 large egg

Directions:

Chili:

1. Heat the olive oil in a large pot over medium heat. Add the onion and garlic, cooking until they start to soften.
2. Add the sweet potato, chili powder, cumin, and cayenne pepper if using. Stir everything together.
3. Add the black beans, diced tomatoes, and vegetable broth. Season with salt and pepper.
4. Bring the mixture to a boil, then reduce the heat and let it simmer for about 30 minutes, or until the sweet potatoes are soft.
5. Adjust the seasonings if needed.

Cornbread:

1. Preheat your oven to 400 degrees F (200 degrees C) and grease a 9-inch round cake pan or cast iron skillet.
2. In a large bowl, combine the cornmeal, flour, sugar, baking powder, and salt.
3. In another bowl, whisk together the milk, vegetable oil, and egg.
4. Pour the wet ingredients into the dry ingredients, stirring until just combined.
5. Pour the batter into the prepared pan.
6. Bake for 20-25 minutes, or until a toothpick inserted into the center comes out clean.
7. Let the cornbread cool for a few minutes before cutting it into slices.

Calories: 500   **Protein:** 17g   **Fat:** 13g   **Carbohydrates:** 84g

6.11 Grilled Chicken Caesar Salad with Whole Grain Croutons

Preparation time: 20 minutes   **Cooking time:** 20 minutes   **Servings:** 4

Ingredients:

For the Salad:

- 4 skinless, boneless chicken breasts
- 2 heads of Romaine lettuce, washed and torn into pieces
- 1/2 cup grated Parmesan cheese
- Salt and pepper to taste

For the Whole Grain Croutons:

- 4 slices whole grain bread, cut into cubes
- 2 tablespoons olive oil
- 1/2 teaspoon garlic powder
- Salt to taste

For the Dressing:

- 2 cloves garlic, minced
- 1 teaspoon Dijon mustard
- 2 tablespoons lemon juice
- 1/2 cup low-fat mayonnaise
- 1/4 cup grated Parmesan cheese
- Salt and pepper to taste

Directions:

1. Preheat your grill to medium-high heat. Season the chicken breasts with salt and pepper, then grill for 6-7 minutes on each side, or until cooked through. Let them rest for a few minutes, then slice.
2. While the chicken is grilling, make the croutons. Preheat your oven to 375 degrees F (190 degrees C). Toss the bread cubes with the olive oil, garlic powder, and salt. Spread them out on a baking sheet and bake for 10-15 minutes, or until golden brown.
3. Make the dressing by whisking together the garlic, Dijon mustard, lemon juice, mayonnaise, and Parmesan cheese. Season with salt and pepper to taste.
4. In a large bowl, combine the lettuce, grilled chicken, croutons, and Parmesan cheese. Toss with the dressing until everything is well coated.

Calories: 450   **Protein:** 40g   **Fat:** 20g   **Carbohydrates:** 24g

6.12 Ground Turkey and Vegetable Stuffed Bell Peppers

Preparation time: 20 minutes   **Cooking time:** 45 minutes   **Servings:** 4

Ingredients:

- 4 large bell peppers (any color)
- 1 lb. ground turkey
- 1 tablespoon olive oil
- 1 medium onion, finely diced
- 2 cloves garlic, minced
- 1 medium zucchini, diced
- 1 medium carrot, diced
- 1 can (14.5 oz.) diced tomatoes (drained)
- 1 teaspoon Italian seasoning or dried basil
- Salt and pepper to taste
- 1 cup cooked brown rice
- 1 cup shredded cheese (cheddar or mozzarella), optional
- Fresh parsley for garnish (optional)

Directions:

1. Preheat oven to 375°F (190°C).
2. Cut off the tops of the bell peppers and remove the seeds. Set aside.
3. In a large skillet, heat olive oil over medium heat. Add onions and garlic, sautéing until translucent.
4. Add ground turkey to the skillet. Cook until browned, breaking it up into small pieces.
5. Add the zucchini, carrot, diced tomatoes, Italian seasoning, salt, and pepper. Continue cooking for another 5-7 minutes, until vegetables are slightly softened.
6. Stir in the cooked brown rice, ensuring that everything is well combined.
7. Stuff each bell pepper with the turkey and vegetable mixture. If using cheese, sprinkle some on top of each filled pepper.
8. Place the stuffed peppers in a baking dish. Add about an inch of water to the bottom of the dish to prevent peppers from drying out.
9. Cover the baking dish with aluminum foil and bake in the preheated oven for about 35-40 minutes, or until the bell peppers are tender.
10. Once done, remove from the oven and allow to cool for a few minutes. Garnish with fresh parsley if desired.

Calories: 320   **Protein:** 28g   **Fat:** 10g   **Carbohydrates:** 28g

6.13 Baked Chicken Thighs with Roasted Root Vegetables

Preparation time: 20 minutes   **Cooking time:** 45 minutes   **Servings:** 4

Ingredients:

- 4 chicken thighs
- 2 tablespoons olive oil
- Salt and pepper to taste
- 1 teaspoon dried rosemary
- 1 teaspoon dried thyme
- 2 large carrots, cut into chunks
- 2 parsnips, cut into chunks
- 2 sweet potatoes, cut into chunks
- 1 red onion, cut into wedges

Directions:

1. Preheat your oven to 400°F (200°C).
2. Rub the chicken thighs with 1 tablespoon of olive oil, then season with salt, pepper, half of the rosemary, and half of the thyme.
3. Place the chicken thighs skin-side up in a large roasting pan.
4. In a separate bowl, toss the chopped vegetables with the remaining olive oil, rosemary, and thyme.
5. Scatter the vegetables around the chicken thighs in the roasting pan.
6. Bake for 45 minutes, or until the chicken is fully cooked and the vegetables are tender and lightly browned. Be sure to turn the vegetables halfway through cooking to ensure even roasting.

Calories: 450   **Protein:** 25g   **Fat:** 25g   **Carbohydrates:** 35g

6.14 Pesto Pasta with Cherry Tomatoes and Grilled Chicken

Preparation time: 15 minutes   **Cooking time:** 20 minutes   **Servings:** 4

Ingredients:

- 2 chicken breasts
- 8 oz whole grain pasta
- Salt and pepper to taste
- 2 tablespoons olive oil
- 1 cup basil pesto (store-bought or homemade)
- 1 cup cherry tomatoes, halved
- Grated Parmesan cheese for serving

Directions:

1. Season the chicken breasts with salt and pepper. Heat 1 tablespoon of olive oil in a grill pan or skillet over medium-high heat. Cook the chicken until it is no longer pink in the middle, about 6-7 minutes per side depending on thickness. Once done, set aside to rest, then slice into strips.
2. While the chicken is cooking, bring a large pot of salted water to a boil. Cook the pasta according to package instructions until al dente. Drain, reserving a cup of pasta water.
3. In the same pot, add the pesto, the remaining olive oil, and a bit of the pasta water. Stir until you have a smooth sauce.
4. Add the cooked pasta back to the pot and toss until it's coated in the pesto sauce. If the sauce is too thick, add more pasta water.
5. Stir in the cherry tomatoes and the grilled chicken strips.
6. Serve hot with a sprinkle of grated Parmesan cheese on top.

Calories: 525   **Protein:** 30g   **Fat:** 20g   **Carbohydrates:** 55g

6.15 Vegan Stuffed Sweet Potatoes with Quinoa and Spinach

Preparation time: 10 minutes   **Cooking time:** 45 minutes   **Servings:** 4

Ingredients:

- 4 medium-sized sweet potatoes
- 1 cup quinoa
- 2 cups vegetable broth or water
- 2 tablespoons olive oil
- 1 small onion, diced
- 2 cloves garlic, minced
- 4 cups fresh spinach
- Salt and pepper to taste
- Optional: Vegan cheese for topping

Directions:

1. Preheat the oven to 400°F (200°C). Prick the sweet potatoes several times with a fork and place them on a baking sheet. Bake for about 45 minutes, or until tender.
2. While the sweet potatoes are baking, prepare the quinoa. Rinse the quinoa under cold water until the water runs clear. Add the quinoa and vegetable broth to a pot. Bring to a boil, then reduce heat to low, cover, and let it simmer for about 15 minutes, or until all the liquid is absorbed.
3. In a large skillet, heat the olive oil over medium heat. Add the diced onion and cook until it becomes translucent. Add the minced garlic and cook for an additional minute.
4. Add the spinach to the skillet and cook until wilted. Season with salt and pepper to taste.
5. Once the quinoa is cooked, add it to the skillet and stir to combine with the spinach mixture.
6. When the sweet potatoes are done, let them cool for a few minutes. Then, cut a slit lengthwise down the middle of each potato. Use a fork to fluff up the insides and create a well for the filling.
7. Stuff each sweet potato with the quinoa and spinach mixture. Top with vegan cheese, if using.
8. Serve the stuffed sweet potatoes warm. Enjoy!

Calories: 410   **Protein:** 12g   **Fat:** 10g   **Carbohydrates:** 67g

7 Snacks and Sides

7.1 Greek Yogurt with Mixed Berries and Honey

Preparation time: 5 minutes   **Cooking time:** 0 minutes   **Servings:** 1

Ingredients:

- 1 cup of Greek yogurt (plain, non-fat)
- 1 cup of mixed berries (strawberries, blueberries, raspberries)
- 1 tablespoon of honey

Directions:

1. Rinse the berries under cold water and pat dry. If you're using strawberries, remove the green tops and cut them in halves or quarters.
2. In a bowl, place the Greek yogurt.
3. Top the yogurt with the mixed berries.
4. Drizzle the honey over the berries and yogurt.
5. You can enjoy it immediately or refrigerate it for later use.

Calories: 220   **Protein:** 23g   **Fat:** 0.5g   **Carbohydrates:** 32g

7.2 Baked Sweet Potato Fries

Preparation time: 10 minutes   **Cooking time:** 30 minutes   **Servings:** 4

Ingredients:

- 2 large sweet potatoes
- 2 tablespoons of olive oil
- 1/2 teaspoon of sea salt
- 1/4 teaspoon of black pepper
- 1/2 teaspoon of paprika

Directions:

1. Preheat your oven to 425°F (220°C) and line a baking sheet with parchment paper.
2. Rinse and dry the sweet potatoes. Cut them into 1/2-inch wide and 3-inch long fries.
3. In a large bowl, combine the cut sweet potatoes, olive oil, salt, pepper, and paprika. Toss until all the fries are well coated.
4. Spread the fries out in a single layer on the prepared baking sheet. Make sure they aren't touching too much to ensure even cooking.
5. Bake for 15 minutes, then take the tray out and flip the fries. Bake for another 15-20 minutes or until they are crispy and golden brown.
6. Remove from the oven and let cool slightly before serving.

Calories: 170   **Protein:** 2g   **Fat:** 7g   **Carbohydrates:** 26g

7.3 Baked Kale Chips

Preparation time: 10 minutes   **Cooking time:** 15 minutes   **Servings:** 4

Ingredients:

- 1 large bunch of kale
- 1 tablespoon olive oil
- 1/4 teaspoon sea salt
- 1/4 teaspoon black pepper
- 1/4 teaspoon garlic powder

Directions:

1. Preheat your oven to 300°F (150°C) and line a baking sheet with parchment paper.
2. Rinse the kale and pat dry completely.
3. Remove the kale leaves from their stems and tear into bite-size pieces.
4. In a large bowl, toss the kale with olive oil. Then season with salt, pepper, and garlic powder, ensuring every leaf is evenly coated.
5. Spread the kale out on your prepared baking sheet. Make sure the leaves are not overlapping.
6. Bake in the preheated oven for about 10-15 minutes, or until the edges of the kale are slightly brown and crispy.
7. Let the chips cool before serving to allow them to crisp up further.

Calories: 60   **Protein:** 2g   **Fat:** 3g   **Carbohydrates:** 7g

7.4 Homemade Hummus with Raw Veggies

Preparation time: 15 minutes   **Cooking time:** 0 minutes   **Servings:** 4

Ingredients:

For the Hummus:

- 1 can (15 oz) chickpeas, drained and rinsed
- 2 cloves of garlic
- 2 tablespoons of tahini
- Juice of 1 lemon
- 2 tablespoons of olive oil
- 1/2 teaspoon of cumin
- Salt to taste
- 2-3 tablespoons of water, or as needed

For the Veggies:

- 2 carrots, peeled and cut into sticks
- 2 bell peppers, cut into strips
- 1 cucumber, cut into sticks

Directions:

1. In a food processor, combine the chickpeas, garlic, tahini, lemon juice, olive oil, cumin, and salt.
2. Process until smooth. If the mixture is too thick, add water one tablespoon at a time until it reaches the desired consistency.
3. Taste and adjust seasonings if necessary.
4. Serve the hummus in a bowl with the raw veggies on the side for dipping.

Calories: 270   **Protein:** 8g   **Fat:** 16g   **Carbohydrates:** 25g

7.5 Fresh Spring Rolls with Peanut Sauce

Preparation time: 30 minutes   **Cooking time:** 0 minutes   **Servings:** 4

Ingredients:

For the Spring Rolls:
- 8 rice paper wrappers
- 2 cups shredded lettuce
- 1 large carrot, julienned
- 1 cucumber, julienned

- 1 bell pepper, thinly sliced
- 1 cup fresh cilantro leaves
- 1 cup fresh mint leaves
- 1 cup cooked, peeled shrimp or tofu for a vegan option (optional)

For the Peanut Sauce:
- 1/3 cup creamy natural peanut butter
- 2 tablespoons soy sauce
- 1 tablespoon honey or maple syrup for vegan

- 1 tablespoon lime juice
- 1-2 tablespoons water to thin, if needed

Directions:

1. Begin with preparing the peanut sauce. In a bowl, mix the peanut butter, soy sauce, honey, lime juice. If the sauce is too thick, add some water to thin. Set aside.
2. To prepare the spring rolls, dip each rice paper wrapper in warm water for a few seconds until it softens up. Place it flat onto your working surface.
3. In the center of the wrapper, place a small amount of lettuce, carrot, cucumber, bell pepper, cilantro, mint, and shrimp or tofu if using.
4. Fold in the sides of the wrapper and roll it up tightly like a burrito. Repeat with the remaining ingredients.
5. Serve the spring rolls with the peanut sauce for dipping.

Calories: 270   **Protein:** 12g   **Fat:** 9g   **Carbohydrates:** 35g

7.6 Carrot and Cucumber Sticks with Ranch Dip

Preparation time: 10 minutes   **Cooking time:** 0 minutes   **Servings:** 4

Ingredients:

- 2 large carrots
- 2 large cucumbers

- 1 cup ranch dressing (preferably low-fat)

Directions:

1. Wash the carrots and cucumbers under cool water to remove any dirt or debris.
2. Peel the carrots and cucumbers if desired, though you may also choose to leave the skin on for extra fiber and nutrients.
3. Cut the carrots and cucumbers into sticks, about 4 inches long and 1/2 inch thick.
4. Arrange the carrot and cucumber sticks on a plate with a bowl of ranch dressing in the middle for dipping.
5. Serve immediately, or refrigerate until ready to serve.

Calories: 180   **Protein:** 1g   **Fat:** 15g   **Carbohydrates:** 9g

7.7 Oven-Roasted Spiced Chickpeas

Preparation time: 10 minutes   **Cooking time:** 20-25 minutes   **Servings:** 4

Ingredients:

- 2 cans (15 ounces each) chickpeas
- 1 tablespoon olive oil
- 1 teaspoon ground cumin
- 1/2 teaspoon smoked paprika
- 1/2 teaspoon garlic powder
- Salt and pepper to taste

Directions:

1. Preheat your oven to 400°F (200°C) and line a baking sheet with parchment paper.
2. Drain and rinse the chickpeas, then dry them thoroughly using a clean dish towel.
3. In a large bowl, toss the chickpeas with the olive oil, cumin, smoked paprika, garlic powder, salt, and pepper until they're well-coated.
4. Spread the chickpeas out evenly on the prepared baking sheet.
5. Bake for 20-25 minutes, or until the chickpeas are crispy and golden. Make sure to give them a good stir halfway through to ensure even roasting.
6. Let the chickpeas cool slightly before serving. They can be enjoyed warm or at room temperature.

Calories: 230   **Protein:** 10g   **Fat:** 6g   **Carbohydrates:** 33g

7.8 Protein-Packed Smoothie Bowl with Granola

Preparation time: 10 minutes   **Cooking time:** 0 minutes   **Servings:** 2

Ingredients:

- 2 bananas, frozen
- 1 cup mixed berries, frozen
- 1 scoop protein powder (vanilla or unflavored)
- 1/2 cup almond milk (or any other non-dairy milk)
- 1/2 cup granola
- Toppings: Fresh fruit, coconut flakes, chia seeds, and a drizzle of honey (optional)

Directions:

1. In a blender, add the frozen bananas, mixed berries, protein powder, and almond milk. Blend until smooth and creamy.
2. Pour the smoothie mixture into two bowls.
3. Top each bowl with granola and your chosen toppings.
4. Serve immediately and enjoy!

Calories: 350   **Protein:** 20g   **Fat:** 8g   **Carbohydrates:** 55g

7.9 Banana and Peanut Butter Smoothie

Preparation time: 5 minutes   **Cooking time:** 0 minutes   **Servings:** 2

Ingredients:

- 2 bananas
- 2 tablespoons natural peanut butter
- 1 cup almond milk (or other non-dairy milk)
- 1 cup ice
- 1 teaspoon honey or other sweetener (optional)
- 1 scoop protein powder (vanilla or unflavored, optional)

Directions:

1. Peel the bananas and place them into your blender.
2. Add the peanut butter, almond milk, ice, and optional honey or protein powder.
3. Blend on high speed until all ingredients are well combined and the smoothie is creamy and smooth.
4. Pour the smoothie into two glasses and serve immediately.

Calories: 275   **Protein:** 8g   **Fat:** 12g   **Carbohydrates:** 38g

7.10 Oven-Roasted Brussels Sprouts

Preparation time: 10 minutes   **Cooking time:** 20-25 minutes   **Servings:** 4

Ingredients:

- 1.5 lbs Brussels sprouts
- 2 tablespoons olive oil
- Salt and pepper to taste
- Optional: 2 cloves of garlic, minced
- Optional: Red pepper flakes to taste

Directions:

1. Preheat your oven to 400°F (200°C) and line a baking sheet with parchment paper.
2. Clean the Brussels sprouts by cutting off the stems and removing any yellow or damaged outer leaves. Cut larger sprouts in half if desired.
3. In a large bowl, toss the Brussels sprouts with olive oil, salt, and pepper. Add the minced garlic and red pepper flakes if using.
4. Spread the Brussels sprouts evenly on the baking sheet, ensuring they aren't overcrowded.
5. Roast in the oven for about 20-25 minutes, or until the Brussels sprouts are tender and caramelized. Stir once or twice during cooking for even roasting.
6. Serve immediately as a side dish with your preferred main course.

Calories: 144   **Protein:** 5g   **Fat:** 8g   **Carbohydrates:** 15g

8 Poultry and Meat Recipes

8.1 Balsamic Glazed Chicken Breast with Roasted Brussels Sprouts

Preparation time: 15 minutes   **Cooking time:** 30 minutes   **Servings:** 4

Ingredients:

For the Chicken:

- 4 boneless skinless chicken breasts
- Salt and pepper to taste
- 1 tablespoon olive oil
- 1/2 cup balsamic vinegar
- 2 tablespoons honey

For the Brussels Sprouts:

- 1 pound Brussels sprouts, trimmed and halved
- 2 tablespoons olive oil
- Salt and pepper to taste

Directions:

1. Preheat your oven to 400°F (200°C). Toss the Brussels sprouts with the olive oil, salt, and pepper and arrange them on a baking sheet. Roast for 20-25 minutes, until golden brown and crispy.
2. While the Brussels sprouts are roasting, season the chicken breasts with salt and pepper. Heat the olive oil in a large skillet over medium heat.
3. Add the chicken breasts and cook for 6-7 minutes on each side, or until cooked through and golden brown.
4. In a small bowl, whisk together the balsamic vinegar and honey. Pour the mixture over the chicken breasts and continue to cook for an additional 2-3 minutes, until the sauce has thickened.
5. Serve the balsamic glazed chicken with the roasted Brussels sprouts on the side.

Calories: 380   **Protein:** 30g   **Fat:** 15g   **Carbohydrates:** 30g

8.2 Baked Chicken Parmesan with Whole Grain Pasta and Marinara Sauce

Preparation time: 15 minutes   **Cooking time:** 30 minutes   **Servings:** 4

Ingredients:

- 4 boneless, skinless chicken breasts (about 1 lb total)
- Salt and black pepper to taste
- 1/2 cup whole wheat bread crumbs
- 1/4 cup grated Parmesan cheese
- 1/2 teaspoon dried basil
- 1/2 teaspoon dried oregano
- 1 tablespoon olive oil
- 2 cups marinara sauce, no added sugar
- 1 cup shredded mozzarella cheese
- 8 oz whole grain spaghetti

Directions:

1. Preheat your oven to 400°F (200°C). Season the chicken breasts on both sides with salt and pepper.
2. In a shallow dish, combine the bread crumbs, Parmesan cheese, basil, and oregano.
3. Dip each chicken breast in the olive oil to coat, then press into the bread crumb mixture.
4. Place the coated chicken breasts in a baking dish. Bake for 20 minutes, or until the chicken is cooked through.
5. While the chicken is baking, cook the whole grain spaghetti according to package instructions.
6. After 20 minutes, remove the chicken from the oven, top each breast with marinara sauce and mozzarella cheese. Return to the oven for an additional 5-10 minutes, until the cheese is melted and bubbly.
7. Serve the chicken over the cooked whole grain spaghetti.

Calories: 430   **Protein:** 40g   **Fat:** 12g   **Carbohydrates:** 40g

8.3 Lemon Garlic Roast Turkey with Sweet Potato Mash

Preparation time: 15 minutes   **Cooking time:** 75 minutes   **Servings:** 4

Ingredients:

- 1.5 lbs turkey breast
- 1 lemon, zested and juiced
- 3 cloves garlic, minced
- 1 tablespoon olive oil
- Salt and pepper to taste
- 4 medium sweet potatoes, peeled and cut into chunks
- 1/4 cup unsweetened almond milk
- 1 tablespoon butter

Directions:

1. Preheat your oven to 375°F (190°C). Place the turkey breast in a roasting pan.
2. In a small bowl, mix together the lemon zest, lemon juice, garlic, olive oil, salt, and pepper. Rub this mixture all over the turkey breast.
3. Roast the turkey in the preheated oven for about 60-75 minutes, or until the internal temperature reaches 165°F (74°C).
4. While the turkey is roasting, place the sweet potatoes in a large pot and cover with water. Bring to a boil, then reduce the heat and simmer for 15-20 minutes, until the sweet potatoes are tender.
5. Drain the sweet potatoes and return them to the pot. Add the almond milk and butter, then mash until smooth. Season with salt and pepper to taste.
6. Once the turkey is done, allow it to rest for a few minutes before slicing. Serve the sliced turkey with the sweet potato mash on the side.

Calories: 400   **Protein:** 48g   **Fat:** 10g   **Carbohydrates:** 35g

8.4 Grilled Tandoori Chicken with Cilantro Mint Chutney

Preparation time: 2 hours 20 minutes   **Cooking time:** 20 minutes   **Servings:** 4

Ingredients:

- 4 boneless, skinless chicken breasts
- 1 cup plain low-fat Greek yogurt
- 2 tablespoons lemon juice
- 1 tablespoon grated fresh ginger
- 2 cloves garlic, minced

For the Cilantro Mint Chutney:

- 1 cup fresh cilantro
- 1/2 cup fresh mint leaves
- 1 green chili, deseeded

- 1 tablespoon garam masala
- 1 teaspoon turmeric
- 1/2 teaspoon cayenne pepper
- Salt to taste
- Fresh cilantro for garnish

- 1 tablespoon lemon juice
- 1/2 teaspoon cumin
- Salt to taste

Directions:

1. In a bowl, mix together the yogurt, lemon juice, ginger, garlic, garam masala, turmeric, cayenne pepper, and salt. Add the chicken breasts and coat them thoroughly with the marinade. Let them marinate in the refrigerator for at least 2 hours, or overnight if possible.
2. Preheat your grill on medium-high heat. Grill the chicken for 7-10 minutes on each side, or until the internal temperature reaches 165°F (74°C).
3. While the chicken is grilling, make the chutney. Combine the cilantro, mint, chili, lemon juice, cumin, and salt in a blender or food processor. Blend until smooth.
4. Serve the grilled chicken with a dollop of cilantro mint chutney and garnish with fresh cilantro.

Calories: 310   **Protein:** 40g   **Fat:** 7g   **Carbohydrates:** 16g

8.5 Slow-Cooked Beef Stew with Root Vegetables

Preparation time: 25 minutes   **Cooking time:** 8 hours   **Servings:** 6

Ingredients:

- 1.5 lbs lean beef stew meat, cut into 1-inch pieces
- 1/2 cup whole wheat flour
- Salt and pepper to taste
- 2 tablespoons olive oil
- 1 onion, chopped
- 3 cloves garlic, minced
- 4 cups low sodium beef broth

- 2 teaspoons Worcestershire sauce
- 2 cups diced carrots
- 2 cups diced parsnips
- 2 cups diced turnips
- 2 cups diced sweet potatoes
- 2 teaspoons fresh thyme leaves
- 2 teaspoons chopped fresh rosemary

Directions:

1. In a large bowl, mix the flour, salt, and pepper. Add the beef and toss to coat.
2. Heat the olive oil in a skillet over medium heat. Add the beef and brown on all sides, then transfer to a slow cooker.
3. In the same skillet, add the onion and garlic, cook until softened. Transfer to the slow cooker.
4. Add the beef broth, Worcestershire sauce, carrots, parsnips, turnips, sweet potatoes, thyme, and rosemary to the slow cooker. Stir to combine.
5. Cover and cook on low for 8 hours or until the beef is tender and the vegetables are cooked through.
6. Adjust the seasoning if necessary and serve warm.

Calories: 350   **Protein:** 32g   **Fat:** 10g   **Carbohydrates:** 35g

8.6 Rosemary Garlic Lamb Chops with Quinoa Salad

Preparation time: 20 minutes   **Cooking time:** 20 minutes   **Servings:** 4

Ingredients:

For the Lamb Chops:

- 8 lamb chops
- 4 cloves garlic, minced
- 2 tablespoons fresh rosemary, chopped
- Salt and pepper to taste
- 2 tablespoons olive oil

For the Quinoa Salad:

- 1 cup quinoa
- 2 cups water
- 1/2 cup cherry tomatoes, halved
- 1 cucumber, diced
- 1/4 cup red onion, finely chopped
- 1/4 cup fresh parsley, chopped
- 2 tablespoons lemon juice
- 2 tablespoons olive oil
- Salt and pepper to taste

Directions:

1. In a large bowl, mix the garlic, rosemary, salt, pepper, and olive oil. Add the lamb chops and turn to coat. Let marinate for at least 15 minutes.
2. Meanwhile, cook the quinoa. Bring the water to a boil, add the quinoa, reduce the heat to low, cover, and cook for 15 minutes. Let sit covered for 5 more minutes then fluff with a fork.
3. Heat a grill pan over medium-high heat. Cook the lamb chops for 4-5 minutes per side or until desired doneness.
4. In a large bowl, combine the cooked quinoa, cherry tomatoes, cucumber, red onion, parsley, lemon juice, olive oil, salt, and pepper. Toss well to combine.
5. Serve the lamb chops with the quinoa salad.

Calories: 500   **Protein:** 35g   **Fat:** 25g   **Carbohydrates:** 35g

8.7 Herb-Roasted Chicken Thighs with Steamed Asparagus

Preparation time: 10 minutes   **Cooking time:** 35 minutes   **Servings:** 4

Ingredients:

- 8 bone-in, skin-on chicken thighs
- 2 tablespoons olive oil
- 2 tablespoons fresh rosemary, chopped
- 2 tablespoons fresh thyme, chopped
- Salt and pepper to taste
- 1 bunch asparagus, trimmed
- 2 tablespoons lemon juice

Directions:

1. Preheat your oven to 425°F (220°C).
2. In a large bowl, mix together the olive oil, rosemary, thyme, salt, and pepper. Add the chicken thighs and toss until they're well coated.
3. Arrange the chicken thighs on a baking sheet, skin side up. Roast in the preheated oven for about 30-35 minutes, or until the chicken is cooked through and the skin is crispy.
4. While the chicken is roasting, steam the asparagus. Fill a pot with a few inches of water and bring it to a boil. Add the asparagus to a steamer basket, season with salt and pepper, and place the basket in the pot. Cover the pot and let the asparagus steam for 5 minutes, or until it's tender.
5. Remove the asparagus from the steamer basket and toss it with the lemon juice.
6. Serve the herb-roasted chicken thighs with the steamed asparagus.

Calories: 450   **Protein:** 38g   **Fat:** 30g   **Carbohydrates:** 5g

8.8 Grilled Turkey Burgers with Sweet Potato Fries

Preparation time: 20 minutes **Cooking time:** 30 minutes **Servings:** 4

Ingredients:

For the Turkey Burgers:

- 1 pound ground turkey
- 1/4 cup whole grain bread crumbs
- 1/4 cup finely chopped onion
- 1 tablespoon chopped fresh parsley
- 1/2 teaspoon salt
- 1/4 teaspoon black pepper
- 4 whole grain hamburger buns
- Lettuce, tomatoes, and pickles for serving

For the Sweet Potato Fries:

- 2 large sweet potatoes, peeled and cut into fries
- 2 tablespoons olive oil
- 1/2 teaspoon paprika
- Salt and pepper to taste

Directions:

1. Preheat your grill to medium heat. While it's heating up, combine the ground turkey, bread crumbs, onion, parsley, salt, and pepper in a large bowl. Mix until everything is well incorporated.
2. Form the mixture into 4 patties and place them on the grill. Cook for about 5-6 minutes on each side, or until the burgers are cooked through.
3. While the burgers are cooking, preheat your oven to 400°F (200°C). Toss the sweet potato fries with the olive oil, paprika, salt, and pepper and arrange them on a baking sheet.
4. Bake for 20-25 minutes, flipping halfway through, until the fries are crispy and golden brown.
5. Serve the turkey burgers on whole grain buns with lettuce, tomatoes, and pickles, alongside the sweet potato fries.

Calories: 450 **Protein:** 32g **Fat:** 18g **Carbohydrates:** 45g

8.9 Baked Chicken Wings with Spicy BBQ Sauce

Preparation time: 15 minutes **Cooking time:** 45 minutes **Servings:** 4

Ingredients:

- 2 lbs chicken wings
- Salt and pepper to taste
- 1 tablespoon olive oil
- 1/2 cup low sodium BBQ sauce
- 1 tablespoon hot sauce (adjust according to your spice preference)

Directions:

1. Preheat your oven to 400°F (200°C). Line a baking sheet with foil for easy clean-up.
2. In a large bowl, toss the chicken wings with the olive oil, salt, and pepper.
3. Arrange the wings in a single layer on the prepared baking sheet.
4. Bake the wings in the preheated oven for 40 minutes, or until they are crispy and fully cooked.
5. While the wings are baking, mix together the BBQ sauce and hot sauce in a small bowl.
6. Remove the wings from the oven and brush them with the spicy BBQ sauce. Return the wings to the oven for another 5 minutes to allow the sauce to caramelize.
7. Serve the wings hot, with extra sauce on the side for dipping if desired.

Calories: 275 **Protein:** 22g **Fat:** 18g **Carbohydrates:** 5g

8.10 Lean Beef and Vegetable Stir Fry with Brown Rice

Preparation time: 20 minutes   **Cooking time:** 20 minutes   **Servings:** 4

Ingredients:

- 1 cup brown rice
- 2 cups water
- 1 pound lean beef strips
- 2 tablespoons olive oil
- 2 garlic cloves, minced
- 1 bell pepper, sliced
- 1 medium carrot, sliced
- 1 zucchini, sliced
- 2 tablespoons low sodium soy sauce
- 2 tablespoons oyster sauce
- Salt and pepper to taste

Directions:

1. Cook the brown rice according to the package instructions. Typically, bring 2 cups of water to a boil, then add the rice, reduce the heat to low, cover and let simmer for 45-50 minutes.
2. While the rice is cooking, heat the olive oil in a large skillet over medium heat. Add the beef strips and cook for 3-4 minutes, or until browned. Remove the beef from the skillet and set aside.
3. In the same skillet, add the minced garlic, bell pepper, carrot, and zucchini. Cook for 5-6 minutes, or until the vegetables are tender.
4. Return the beef to the skillet and add the soy sauce and oyster sauce. Stir to combine and cook for an additional 2-3 minutes, until the beef is cooked through and the sauce is heated.
5. Serve the beef and vegetable stir fry over the cooked brown rice.

Calories: 420   **Protein:** 30g   **Fat:** 12g   **Carbohydrates:** 50g

9 Fish and Seafood Recipes

9.1 Baked Cod with Tomatoes and Olives

Preparation time: 10 minutes   **Cooking time:** 20 minutes   **Servings:** 4

Ingredients:

- 4 cod fillets (about 6 ounces each)
- Salt and pepper to taste
- 2 tablespoons olive oil
- 1 onion, thinly sliced
- 2 cloves garlic, minced
- 1 can (14.5 ounces) diced tomatoes
- 1/2 cup pitted Kalamata olives
- 1 teaspoon dried basil
- 1/2 teaspoon dried oregano
- Fresh basil leaves for garnish

Directions:

1. Preheat the oven to 400°F (200°C).
2. Season the cod fillets with salt and pepper and place them in a baking dish.
3. Heat the olive oil in a large skillet over medium heat. Add the onion and garlic and cook until softened, about 5 minutes.
4. Stir in the diced tomatoes, Kalamata olives, dried basil, and dried oregano. Simmer for a few minutes until the flavors are combined.
5. Pour the tomato and olive mixture over the cod fillets.
6. Bake in the preheated oven for about 15 minutes, or until the cod is cooked through and flakes easily with a fork.
7. Garnish with fresh basil leaves before serving.

Calories: 260   **Protein:** 28g   **Fat:** 10g   **Carbohydrates:** 14g

9.2 Pan-Seared Scallops with Lemon Garlic Pasta

Preparation time: 10 minutes   **Cooking time:** 20 minutes   **Servings:** 4

Ingredients:

- 1 pound of scallops
- Salt and pepper to taste
- 2 tablespoons olive oil
- 2 cloves garlic, minced
- Zest and juice of 1 lemon
- 2 cups whole grain spaghetti, cooked according to package instructions
- 1/4 cup fresh parsley, chopped
- Red pepper flakes to taste (optional)

Directions:

1. Pat the scallops dry with paper towels, then season with salt and pepper.
2. Heat the olive oil in a large skillet over medium-high heat. Add the scallops and sear until golden brown, about 2 minutes per side. Remove the scallops from the skillet and set aside.
3. In the same skillet, add the minced garlic, lemon zest, and lemon juice. Cook for a minute until the garlic is fragrant.
4. Add the cooked spaghetti to the skillet and toss to combine with the lemon garlic sauce.
5. Return the scallops to the skillet and toss gently to combine with the pasta.
6. Sprinkle with chopped parsley and red pepper flakes (if using) before serving.

Calories: 370   **Protein:** 25g   **Fat:** 8g   **Carbohydrates:** 50g

9.3 Panko-Crusted Tilapia with Steamed Veggies

Preparation time: 15 minutes   **Cooking time:** 20 minutes   **Servings:** 4

Ingredients:

- 4 tilapia fillets
- 1 cup panko breadcrumbs
- 1 teaspoon paprika
- Salt and pepper to taste
- 2 tablespoons olive oil
- 1 large head broccoli, cut into florets
- 2 large carrots, peeled and sliced
- 1 red bell pepper, cut into strips
- Lemon wedges, for serving

Directions:

1. Preheat your oven to 400°F (200°C) and line a baking sheet with parchment paper.
2. In a shallow bowl, mix together the panko breadcrumbs, paprika, salt, and pepper.
3. Brush each tilapia fillet with a bit of olive oil, then press it into the breadcrumb mixture to coat both sides. Place the fillets on the prepared baking sheet.
4. Bake the tilapia for 15-20 minutes, or until the fish flakes easily with a fork.
5. While the fish is baking, steam the broccoli, carrots, and bell pepper until they're tender-crisp. You can do this in a steamer basket over boiling water, or in the microwave with a bit of water.
6. Serve the baked tilapia with the steamed veggies on the side, and a lemon wedge for squeezing over top.

Calories: 350   **Protein:** 28g   **Fat:** 12g   **Carbohydrates:** 30g

9.4 Seafood Paella with Brown Rice

Preparation time: 20 minutes   **Cooking time:** 40 minutes   **Servings:** 4

Ingredients:

- 1 cup brown rice
- 2 cups low-sodium chicken broth
- 1 tablespoon olive oil
- 1 medium onion, chopped
- 3 cloves garlic, minced
- 1 red bell pepper, chopped
- 1 teaspoon paprika
- 1/2 teaspoon turmeric
- 1/4 teaspoon cayenne pepper
- 1/2 pound shrimp, peeled and deveined
- 1/2 pound mussels, scrubbed and de-bearded
- 1/2 pound calamari rings
- 1/2 cup frozen peas, thawed
- Salt and pepper to taste
- Lemon wedges, for serving

Directions:

1. Rinse the brown rice under cold water until the water runs clear. Combine the rinsed rice and chicken broth in a saucepan. Bring to a boil, then reduce heat to low, cover, and let simmer for about 45 minutes, or until the rice is tender and the liquid is absorbed.
2. While the rice is cooking, heat the olive oil in a large skillet over medium heat. Add the onion, garlic, and bell pepper. Cook until the vegetables are softened, about 5 minutes.
3. Stir in the paprika, turmeric, and cayenne pepper. Add the shrimp, mussels, and calamari. Cook until the shrimp are pink and the mussels have opened, about 5-7 minutes
4. Once the rice is cooked, stir it into the seafood mixture along with the peas. Cook for another few minutes until everything is heated through. Season with salt and pepper to taste.
5. Serve the paella with lemon wedges on the side.

Calories: 350   **Protein:** 28g   **Fat:** 6g   **Carbohydrates:** 45g

9.5 Asian-Inspired Shrimp Stir Fry with Brown Rice

Preparation time: 15 minutes   **Cooking time:** 20 minutes   **Servings:** 4

Ingredients:

- 1 cup uncooked brown rice
- 2 cups water
- 1 tablespoon olive oil
- 1 pound large shrimp, peeled and deveined
- 2 cloves garlic, minced
- 1 onion, sliced
- 1 bell pepper, sliced
- 1 zucchini, sliced
- 1 cup snap peas
- 2 tablespoons low-sodium soy sauce
- 1 tablespoon oyster sauce
- 1 teaspoon cornstarch, mixed with 1 tablespoon cold water
- 1 teaspoon sesame seeds (for garnish)

Directions:

1. Start by cooking the brown rice according to the package instructions. Generally, you'll bring the water to a boil, add the rice, then reduce to a simmer, cover, and let it cook for about 45 minutes, or until the water is absorbed and the rice is tender.
2. While the rice is cooking, heat the olive oil in a large pan or wok over medium-high heat.
3. Add the shrimp and cook until pink, about 2-3 minutes per side. Remove the shrimp from the pan and set aside.
4. In the same pan, add the garlic, onion, bell pepper, zucchini, and snap peas. Stir fry for about 5 minutes, or until the vegetables are tender-crisp.
5. Return the shrimp to the pan. Stir in the soy sauce, oyster sauce, and cornstarch-water mixture. Continue to stir fry for another 2-3 minutes, until the sauce has thickened.
6. Serve the shrimp stir fry over the cooked brown rice, garnished with sesame seeds.

Calories: 350   **Protein:** 25g   **Fat:** 6g   **Carbohydrates:** 49g

9.6 Oven-Baked Trout with Herbs and Lemon

Preparation time: 10 minutes   **Cooking time:** 15 minutes   **Servings:** 4

Ingredients:

- 4 trout fillets
- 2 tablespoons olive oil
- 1 lemon, sliced
- 2 cloves garlic, minced
- 1 tablespoon fresh dill, chopped
- 1 tablespoon fresh parsley, chopped
- Salt and black pepper to taste

Directions:

1. Preheat your oven to 400 degrees F (200 degrees C) and line a baking tray with aluminum foil.
2. Lay the trout fillets skin-side-down on the tray. Drizzle with olive oil and season with salt and pepper.
3. Sprinkle the minced garlic, chopped dill, and chopped parsley evenly over the trout fillets.
4. Lay the lemon slices on top of the fillets.
5. Bake in the preheated oven for 10-15 minutes, or until the trout is cooked through and flakes easily with a fork.

Calories: 275   **Protein:** 35g   **Fat:** 13g   **Carbohydrates:** 2g

9.7 Lobster Salad with Avocado and Grapefruit

Preparation time: 20 minutes   **Cooking time:** 20 minutes   **Servings:** 4

Ingredients:

- 2 cooked lobsters, meat removed and chopped
- 2 avocados, peeled, pitted, and diced
- 2 grapefruits, segmented
- 4 cups mixed salad greens
- 1/4 cup olive oil
- 2 tablespoons freshly squeezed lemon juice
- Salt and black pepper to taste

Directions:

1. Place the chopped lobster meat, diced avocados, and segmented grapefruit in a large bowl. Toss gently to combine.
2. In a small bowl, whisk together the olive oil and lemon juice. Season with salt and pepper.
3. Drizzle the dressing over the lobster mixture. Toss gently to ensure everything is well coated.
4. Divide the mixed greens among 4 plates. Top with the lobster mixture.
5. Serve immediately, and enjoy your refreshing and hearty salad!

Calories: 350   **Protein:** 22g   **Fat:** 24g   **Carbohydrates:** 12g

9.8 Halibut Steaks with Capers and Rosemary

Preparation time: 10 minutes   **Cooking time:** 20 minutes   **Servings:** 4

Ingredients:

- 4 halibut steaks, about 6 ounces each
- 2 tablespoons olive oil
- 2 cloves garlic, minced
- 1 tablespoon fresh rosemary, finely chopped
- 2 tablespoons capers, drained
- Salt and black pepper to taste
- Lemon wedges, for serving

Directions:

1. Preheat your oven to 375°F (190°C).
2. Place the halibut steaks in a baking dish. Drizzle with olive oil and sprinkle with minced garlic, rosemary, capers, salt, and pepper.
3. Place the baking dish in the oven and bake for 15-20 minutes, or until the halibut flakes easily with a fork.
4. Remove from the oven and serve hot with lemon wedges on the side.

Calories: 240   **Protein:** 35g   **Fat:** 10g   **Carbohydrates:** 1g

9.9 Cajun-Spiced Catfish with Collard Greens

Preparation time: 15 minutes   **Cooking time:** 20 minutes   **Servings:** 4

Ingredients:

- 4 catfish fillets
- 2 tablespoons Cajun seasoning
- 1 tablespoon olive oil
- 1 onion, chopped
- 2 cloves garlic, minced
- 1 pound collard greens, stems removed and leaves chopped
- 1 cup low-sodium chicken broth
- Salt and black pepper to taste
- Lemon wedges, for serving

Directions:

1. Season both sides of the catfish fillets with the Cajun seasoning.
2. Heat the olive oil in a large skillet over medium heat. Add the catfish fillets and cook until golden brown and cooked through, about 4-5 minutes per side. Remove the catfish from the skillet and set aside.
3. In the same skillet, add the onion and garlic and cook until softened, about 5 minutes. Add the collard greens, chicken broth, salt, and pepper to the skillet and stir to combine. Cover the skillet and cook until the collard greens are tender, about 10 minutes.
4. Serve the Cajun-spiced catfish with the collard greens and a squeeze of lemon juice.

Calories: 350   **Protein:** 35g   **Fat:** 15g   **Carbohydrates:** 10g

9.10 Clam Chowder with Whole Grain Bread

Preparation time: 15 minutes   **Cooking time:** 45 minutes   **Servings:** 6

Ingredients:

- 2 tablespoons olive oil
- 1 medium onion, diced
- 2 celery stalks, diced
- 2 carrots, peeled and diced
- 2 cloves garlic, minced
- 1.5 pounds of potatoes, peeled and diced
- 1 cup clam juice
- 4 cups low sodium chicken broth
- 2 cans (6.5 ounces each) chopped clams in juice, undrained
- 1 cup fat-free half and half
- Salt and black pepper to taste
- Chopped fresh parsley, for garnish
- 6 slices of whole grain bread

Directions:

1. Heat the olive oil in a large pot over medium heat. Add the onion, celery, carrots, and garlic, and sauté until the vegetables are softened, about 5 minutes.
2. Add the potatoes, clam juice, and chicken broth to the pot. Bring the mixture to a boil, then reduce the heat and simmer until the potatoes are tender, about 20 minutes.
3. Add the chopped clams in their juice to the pot and stir to combine. Cook for another 5 minutes, until the clams are heated through.
4. Stir in the half and half, then season with salt and pepper to taste. Cook for another 5 minutes, until the chowder is heated through.
5. Ladle the chowder into bowls, garnish with fresh parsley, and serve with a slice of whole grain bread on the side.

Calories: 380   **Protein:** 20g   **Fat:** 8g   **Carbohydrates:** 55g

10 Vegetarian and Vegan Recipes

10.1 Spicy Lentil and Vegetable Curry

Preparation time: 15 minutes   **Cooking time:** 40 minutes   **Servings:** 4

Ingredients:

- 1 cup dried lentils
- 1 large onion, chopped
- 2 cloves garlic, minced
- 1 tablespoon fresh ginger, minced
- 1 tablespoon curry powder
- 1 teaspoon turmeric
- 1/2 teaspoon cayenne pepper (or to taste)
- 1 large carrot, diced
- 1 bell pepper, diced
- 1 zucchini, diced
- 1 can diced tomatoes (14.5 oz)
- 3 cups vegetable broth
- 2 cups fresh spinach leaves
- Salt to taste
- 2 tablespoons olive oil
- Fresh cilantro, chopped (for garnish)

Directions:

1. Rinse lentils under cold water until water runs clear.
2. In a large pot, heat olive oil over medium heat. Add onions, garlic, and ginger and sauté until onions become translucent.
3. Add curry powder, turmeric, and cayenne pepper to the pot and cook for another minute until spices are fragrant.
4. Add diced carrot, bell pepper, zucchini, canned tomatoes with their juice, and vegetable broth to the pot. Stir well to combine.
5. Add rinsed lentils to the pot, stir again. Bring the mixture to a boil.
6. Reduce heat, cover the pot, and let it simmer for about 25-30 minutes, or until the lentils and vegetables are tender.
7. Add spinach leaves and salt, stir well. Cook for another 2-3 minutes until spinach is wilted.
8. Serve the curry hot, garnished with chopped fresh cilantro.

Calories: 315   **Protein:** 17g   **Fat:** 9g   **Carbohydrates:** 45g

10.2 Quinoa Stuffed Bell Peppers

Preparation time: 20 minutes   **Cooking time:** 40 minutes   **Servings:** 4

Ingredients:

- 4 large bell peppers (any color)
- 1 cup quinoa, rinsed and drained
- 2 cups vegetable broth
- 1 medium onion, diced
- 2 cloves garlic, minced
- 1 zucchini, diced
- 1 can (15 oz) black beans, rinsed and drained
- 1 can (14.5 oz) diced tomatoes, drained
- 1 tsp olive oil
- 1 tsp cumin
- 1/2 tsp smoked paprika
- 1/4 tsp black pepper
- Salt, to taste
- Fresh parsley or cilantro, chopped (for garnish)
- Optional: Grated cheese (for a non-vegan version)

Directions:

1. Preheat oven to 375°F (190°C).
2. In a medium saucepan, bring the vegetable broth to a boil. Add quinoa, cover, and reduce heat. Simmer for 15 minutes, or until quinoa is cooked and liquid is absorbed. Remove from heat and fluff with a fork.
3. While the quinoa is cooking, cut off the tops of the bell peppers and remove the seeds.
4. In a large skillet, heat olive oil over medium heat. Add onions and garlic, sautéing until translucent.
5. Add diced zucchini to the skillet and cook until softened.
6. Stir in the beans, diced tomatoes, cumin, smoked paprika, salt, and pepper. Mix well and cook for another 5 minutes.
7. Mix the quinoa into the skillet, stirring well to combine all ingredients.
8. Fill each bell pepper with the quinoa mixture and place them in a baking dish. Cover with aluminum foil.
9. Bake in the preheated oven for about 25 minutes, until the peppers are tender.
10. (Optional) Remove foil, top each pepper with grated cheese, and bake for an additional 5-10 minutes, until cheese is melted.
11. Remove from oven, let cool slightly, and garnish with chopped parsley or cilantro before serving.

Calories: 280   **Protein:** 11g   **Fat:** 3.5g   **Carbohydrates:** 52g

10.3 Vegan Sweet Potato and Black Bean Enchiladas

Preparation time: 25 minutes   **Cooking time:** 25 minutes   **Servings:** 4

Ingredients:

- 2 medium sweet potatoes, peeled and diced
- 1 can (15 oz) black beans, rinsed and drained
- 1 cup corn kernels, frozen or fresh
- 1 small onion, chopped
- 2 cloves garlic, minced
- 1 tsp cumin
- 1/2 tsp chili powder
- Salt and pepper to taste
- 8 whole wheat tortillas
- 2 cups enchilada sauce
- 1 ripe avocado, sliced
- Fresh cilantro, chopped (for garnish)

Directions:

1. Preheat your oven to 375°F (190°C).
2. In a medium saucepan, bring water to a boil. Add diced sweet potatoes and cook until tender, about 10-12 minutes. Drain and set aside.
3. In a large skillet over medium heat, sauté the onion and garlic until the onion becomes translucent.
4. Add the cooked sweet potatoes, black beans, corn, cumin, chili powder, salt, and pepper. Stir well to combine.
5. Pour a thin layer of enchilada sauce in the bottom of a baking dish.
6. Divide the sweet potato and black bean mixture evenly among the tortillas, rolling each up tightly and placing them seam-side down in the baking dish.
7. Pour the remaining enchilada sauce over the top of the tortillas. Cover the baking dish with aluminum foil.
8. Bake for 20 minutes, or until heated through.
9. Remove from the oven and top with sliced avocado and fresh cilantro before serving.

Calories: 380   **Protein:** 12g   **Fat:** 8g   **Carbohydrates:** 65g

10.4 Chickpea and Vegetable Stir Fry with Brown Rice

Preparation time: 15 minutes   **Cooking time:** 20 minutes   **Servings:** 4

Ingredients:

- 1 cup brown rice
- 2 cups water
- 1 can chickpeas, drained and rinsed
- 1 tablespoon olive oil
- 1 onion, sliced
- 1 red bell pepper, sliced
- 1 green bell pepper, sliced
- 2 cloves garlic, minced
- 1 tablespoon soy sauce (use a low-sodium version if necessary)
- 1 tablespoon sesame oil
- Salt and pepper to taste
- Sesame seeds for garnish

Directions:

1. Cook the brown rice according to the package instructions, using water. Set aside.
2. While the rice is cooking, heat the olive oil in a large pan over medium heat. Add the onions and bell peppers, and sauté until they start to soften, about 5 minutes.
3. Add the chickpeas and garlic to the pan, and stir to combine. Sauté for another 5 minutes, until the chickpeas are heated through and the garlic is fragrant.
4. Stir in the soy sauce and sesame oil, and season with salt and pepper. Cook for another minute or two, until everything is well combined and heated through.
5. Serve the stir fry over the cooked brown rice, garnished with sesame seeds.

Calories: 345   **Protein:** 12g   **Fat:** 9g   **Carbohydrates:** 55g

10.5 Baked Falafel with Tzatziki Sauce

Preparation time: 15 minutes   **Cooking time:** 20-25 minutes   **Servings:** 4

Ingredients:

- 1 can (15 oz) chickpeas, rinsed and drained
- 1/2 large onion, roughly chopped
- 2 tablespoons fresh parsley, chopped
- 2 tablespoons fresh cilantro, chopped
- 1 teaspoon lemon juice
- 1 teaspoon olive oil

- 1 teaspoon cumin
- 1/2 teaspoon dried red pepper flakes
- 2 cloves of garlic, minced
- 2 tablespoons whole wheat flour
- 1/2 teaspoon baking powder
- Salt to taste

For the Tzatziki Sauce:
- 1 cup Greek yogurt
- 1 cucumber, finely chopped
- 1 tablespoon lemon juice

- 2 cloves garlic, minced
- Salt to taste

Directions:

1. Preheat your oven to 375°F (190°C) and line a baking sheet with parchment paper.
2. In a food processor, combine the chickpeas, onion, parsley, cilantro, lemon juice, olive oil, cumin, red pepper flakes, garlic, and salt. Process until smooth but still slightly chunky.
3. Add in the whole wheat flour and baking powder and pulse a few more times.
4. Shape the mixture into small balls, about 1 inch in diameter, and place them on the prepared baking sheet.
5. Bake for 20-25 minutes, or until the falafel are golden brown and crispy on the outside.
6. While the falafel are baking, make the tzatziki sauce by combining the Greek yogurt, cucumber, lemon juice, garlic, and salt in a small bowl.
7. Serve the falafel warm with the tzatziki sauce on the side.

Calories: 320   **Protein:** 16g   **Fat:** 5g   **Carbohydrates:** 52g

10.6 Vegan Pad Thai with Tofu

Preparation time: 15 minutes   **Cooking time:** 20 minutes   **Servings:** 4

Ingredients:

- 8 ounces rice noodles
- 1 block (14 ounces) firm tofu, drained and cut into cubes
- 2 tablespoons olive oil
- 3 cloves garlic, minced
- 1 red bell pepper, thinly sliced

For the Sauce:

- 3 tablespoons low-sodium soy sauce or tamari
- 1 tablespoon tamarind paste

- 1 cup bean sprouts
- 1/2 cup crushed peanuts
- 1 lime, cut into wedges
- Fresh cilantro, for garnish

- 1 tablespoon agave nectar
- 1/2 teaspoon crushed red pepper flakes (optional)

Directions:

1. Soak the rice noodles in warm water for 10 minutes, then drain and set aside.
2. In a large pan, heat the olive oil over medium heat. Add the tofu cubes and cook until they are golden brown on all sides, about 10 minutes. Remove the tofu from the pan and set aside.
3. In the same pan, add the garlic and red bell pepper, and sauté for about 5 minutes until the pepper is tender.
4. In a small bowl, whisk together the soy sauce or tamari, tamarind paste, agave nectar, and red pepper flakes if using.
5. Add the drained noodles to the pan with the vegetables, pour the sauce over the top, and toss to combine. Cook for a few minutes until the noodles are tender.
6. Add the tofu back to the pan and toss to combine. Stir in the bean sprouts.
7. Serve the pad thai garnished with the crushed peanuts, lime wedges, and fresh cilantro.

Calories: 480   **Protein:** 18g   **Fat:** 16g   **Carbohydrates:** 66g

10.7 Eggplant and Chickpea Stew

Preparation time: 20 minutes   **Cooking time:** 45 minutes   **Servings:** 6

Ingredients:

- 2 tablespoons olive oil
- 1 large onion, chopped
- 3 cloves garlic, minced
- 2 medium eggplants, cubed
- 1 can chickpeas, drained and rinsed
- 1 can diced tomatoes

- 2 cups vegetable broth
- 1 teaspoon cumin
- 1 teaspoon coriander
- Salt and pepper to taste
- Fresh parsley for garnish

Directions:

1. Heat the olive oil in a large pot over medium heat. Add the onion and garlic, and sauté until the onion is translucent, about 5 minutes.
2. Add the eggplant to the pot, and stir to combine. Cook until the eggplant starts to soften, about 10 minutes.
3. Stir in the chickpeas, diced tomatoes, vegetable broth, cumin, and coriander. Season with salt and pepper.
4. Bring the mixture to a simmer, then reduce the heat to low and cover the pot. Let it simmer for about 30 minutes, until the eggplant is completely tender and the flavors have melded together.
5. Serve the stew hot, garnished with fresh parsley.

Calories: 210   **Protein:** 7g   **Fat:** 7g   **Carbohydrates:** 31g

10.8 Lentil Shepherd's Pie

Preparation time: 20 minutes   **Cooking time:** 40 minutes   **Servings:** 6

Ingredients:

- 1 cup green or brown lentils
- 2 cups vegetable broth
- 1 tablespoon olive oil
- 1 onion, diced
- 2 carrots, diced
- 2 cloves garlic, minced

- 1 teaspoon thyme
- 1 teaspoon rosemary
- 2 tablespoons tomato paste
- 1 cup frozen peas
- Salt and pepper to taste

For the Mashed Potatoes:

- 2 large russet potatoes, peeled and diced
- 1/4 cup almond milk

- 2 tablespoons vegan butter
- Salt and pepper to taste

Directions:

1. Rinse the lentils, then add them to a pot with the vegetable broth. Bring to a boil, then reduce the heat and simmer until the lentils are tender and most of the liquid has been absorbed, about 20 minutes.
2. Meanwhile, in a large skillet, heat the olive oil over medium heat. Add the onion, carrots, and garlic, and sauté until the onions are translucent and the carrots are tender, about 10 minutes.
3. Stir in the thyme, rosemary, tomato paste, and peas. Add the cooked lentils and stir to combine. Season with salt and pepper to taste.

4. Preheat your oven to 400°F (200°C).
5. For the mashed potatoes, add the diced potatoes to a pot and cover with water. Bring to a boil, then reduce the heat and simmer until the potatoes are tender, about 15 minutes. Drain, then add the almond milk, vegan butter, salt, and pepper, and mash until smooth.
6. Spread the lentil mixture in a baking dish, then top with the mashed potatoes.
7. Bake for 20 minutes, or until the mashed potatoes are golden on top.

Calories: 280   **Protein:** 12g   **Fat:** 6g   **Carbohydrates:** 48g

10.9 Cauliflower and Potato Curry

Preparation time: 15 minutes **Cooking time:** 40 minutes   **Servings:** 6

Ingredients:

- 1 large cauliflower, cut into florets
- 3 medium potatoes, cubed
- 1 large onion, diced
- 2 cloves garlic, minced
- 1 tablespoon grated ginger
- 1 can diced tomatoes
- 1 cup vegetable broth
- 2 teaspoons curry powder
- 1 teaspoon turmeric
- 1 teaspoon cumin
- Salt and pepper to taste
- 2 tablespoons olive oil
- Fresh cilantro for garnish

Directions:

1. Heat the olive oil in a large pan over medium heat. Add the onion, garlic, and ginger, and sauté until the onion becomes translucent.
2. Add the curry powder, turmeric, and cumin to the pan, and stir well to combine. Cook for another 2 minutes to toast the spices.
3. Add the cauliflower and potatoes to the pan, and stir to coat in the spice mixture.
4. Add the diced tomatoes and vegetable broth to the pan, and season with salt and pepper. Stir well to combine all ingredients.
5. Cover the pan and reduce the heat to low. Simmer for 30 minutes, or until the cauliflower and potatoes are tender.
6. Serve the curry hot, garnished with fresh cilantro.

Calories: 220   **Protein:** 6g   **Fat:** 5g   **Carbohydrates:** 38g

10.10   Mushroom and Spinach Lasagna

Preparation time: 25 minutes **Cooking time:** 45 minutes   **Servings:** 6

Ingredients:

- 9 whole grain lasagna noodles
- 2 cups chopped fresh spinach
- 2 cups sliced mushrooms
- 1 onion, chopped
- 2 cloves garlic, minced
- 1 can (15 ounces) no-salt-added tomato sauce
- 2 cups low-fat ricotta cheese
- 1 cup shredded mozzarella cheese
- 2 tablespoons olive oil
- Salt and pepper to taste

Directions:

1. Preheat your oven to 375°F (190°C). Cook the lasagna noodles according to the package instructions, then drain and set aside.
2. Heat the olive oil in a large pan over medium heat. Add the onion, garlic, and mushrooms, and sauté until the onions are translucent and the mushrooms have released their liquid.
3. Add the spinach to the pan and cook until it's wilted. Remove the pan from the heat and set aside.
4. Spread a layer of tomato sauce on the bottom of a baking dish. Place three lasagna noodles on top of the sauce, then spread a layer of the spinach and mushroom mixture on top. Spread a layer of ricotta cheese on top of the vegetables.
5. Repeat the layers two more times, ending with a layer of tomato sauce. Sprinkle the mozzarella cheese on top.
6. Cover the baking dish with aluminum foil and bake for 30 minutes. Then remove the foil and bake for an additional 15 minutes, or until the cheese is bubbly and golden.
7. Let the lasagna cool for a few minutes before serving.

Calories: 300   **Protein:** 18g   **Fat:** 10g   **Carbohydrates:** 32g

10.11 Vegan Lentil and Vegetable Loaf

Preparation time: 20 minutes   **Cooking time:** 60 minutes   **Servings:** 8

Ingredients:

- 2 cups cooked green lentils
- 1 cup rolled oats
- 1 cup finely chopped vegetables (carrots, celery, bell peppers)
- 1 onion, finely chopped
- 2 cloves of garlic, minced
- 1 can (15 ounces) unsalted diced tomatoes, drained
- 2 tablespoons tomato paste
- 2 tablespoons olive oil
- 1 tablespoon soy sauce
- 1 teaspoon dried thyme
- 1 teaspoon dried oregano
- Salt and pepper to taste

Directions:

1. Preheat your oven to 375°F (190°C). Grease a loaf pan and set it aside.
2. Heat the olive oil in a large pan over medium heat. Add the onion, garlic, and chopped vegetables, and sauté until the vegetables are tender.
3. In a large bowl, combine the cooked lentils, sautéed vegetables, drained tomatoes, oats, tomato paste, soy sauce, thyme, oregano, and a pinch of salt and pepper. Mix until everything is well combined.
4. Transfer the lentil mixture to the prepared loaf pan, pressing it down firmly.
5. Bake for about 60 minutes, or until the top is browned and the loaf is firm.
6. Allow the loaf to cool for a few minutes before removing it from the pan. Slice and serve.

Calories: 220   **Protein:** 12g   **Fat:** 6g   **Carbohydrates:** 30g

10.12   Stuffed Zucchini with Quinoa and Black Beans

Preparation time: 20 minutes   **Cooking time:** 40 minutes   **Servings:** 4

Ingredients:

- 4 large zucchinis
- 1 cup cooked quinoa
- 1 can (15 ounces) black beans, drained and rinsed
- 1 red bell pepper, finely diced
- 1 onion, finely diced
- 2 cloves garlic, minced
- 1 teaspoon ground cumin
- 1/2 teaspoon chili powder
- 2 tablespoons olive oil
- Salt and pepper to taste

Directions:

1. Preheat your oven to 375°F (190°C). Cut the zucchinis in half lengthwise and scoop out the pulp, leaving a shell about 1/4 inch thick. Set aside.
2. Heat the olive oil in a pan over medium heat. Add the onion, garlic, and bell pepper and sauté until they are soft.
3. Add the black beans, quinoa, cumin, chili powder, and a pinch of salt and pepper. Stir until everything is well combined.
4. Spoon the quinoa and black bean mixture into the zucchini halves.
5. Place the stuffed zucchinis on a baking sheet and bake for about 20-25 minutes, until the zucchinis are tender.
6. Serve warm.

Calories: 280   **Protein:** 11g   **Fat:** 8g   **Carbohydrates:** 45g

10.13   Vegetarian Chili with Whole Grain Cornbread

Preparation time: 20 minutes   **Cooking time:** 1 hour   **Servings:** 6

Ingredients:

For the Vegetarian Chili:

- 2 tablespoons olive oil
- 1 large onion, diced
- 2 bell peppers, diced
- 3 cloves garlic, minced
- 2 cans (15 ounces each) kidney beans, drained and rinsed
- 1 can (15 ounces) black beans, drained and rinsed

- 1 can (28 ounces) crushed tomatoes
- 2 tablespoons chili powder
- 1 teaspoon cumin
- 1 teaspoon oregano
- Salt and pepper to taste

For the Whole Grain Cornbread:

- 1 cup whole grain cornmeal
- 1 cup whole wheat flour
- 4 teaspoons baking powder
- 1/4 cup honey

- 1 cup milk
- 1 egg
- 1/4 cup unsalted butter, melted

Directions:

For the Vegetarian Chili:

1. Heat olive oil in a large pot over medium heat. Add the onions, bell peppers, and garlic, and cook until softened, about 5 minutes.
2. Add the kidney beans, black beans, crushed tomatoes, chili powder, cumin, oregano, salt, and pepper. Stir well to combine.

3. Reduce the heat to low, cover the pot, and let the chili simmer for about 45 minutes, stirring occasionally.

For the Whole Grain Cornbread:

1. While the chili is simmering, preheat your oven to 425°F (220°C) and grease a 9-inch baking pan.
2. In a large bowl, combine the cornmeal, flour, and baking powder. In a separate bowl, whisk together the honey, milk, egg, and melted butter. Pour the wet ingredients into the dry ingredients and stir until just combined.
3. Pour the batter into the prepared baking pan and smooth the top with a spatula.

4. Bake for 20-25 minutes, until a toothpick inserted into the center of the cornbread comes out clean.
5. Let the cornbread cool for a few minutes before slicing.

Serve a bowl of the vegetarian chili with a slice of the whole grain cornbread on the side.

Calories: 550   **Protein:** 20g   **Fat:** 12g   **Carbohydrates:** 95g

10.14   Baked Sweet Potato with Vegan Chili

Preparation time: 20 minutes   **Cooking time:** 1 hour   **Servings:** 4

Ingredients:

For the Baked Sweet Potatoes:

- 4 medium-sized sweet potatoes

For the Vegan Chili:

- 1 tablespoon olive oil
- 1 onion, chopped
- 2 cloves garlic, minced
- 1 bell pepper, diced
- 1 can (15 ounces) black beans, drained and rinsed
- 1 can (15 ounces) kidney beans, drained and rinsed
- 1 can (15 ounces) diced tomatoes
- 1 cup vegetable broth
- 2 tablespoons chili powder
- 1 teaspoon cumin
- 1 teaspoon oregano
- Salt and pepper to taste

Directions:

For the Baked Sweet Potatoes:

1. Preheat your oven to 400°F (200°C) and line a baking sheet with parchment paper.
2. Prick each sweet potato several times with a fork and place them on the baking sheet.
3. Bake for 45-50 minutes, or until the sweet potatoes are tender.

For the Vegan Chili:

1. While the sweet potatoes are baking, heat the olive oil in a large pot over medium heat.
2. Add the onion, garlic, and bell pepper, and cook until the vegetables are softened, about 5 minutes.
3. Add the black beans, kidney beans, diced tomatoes, vegetable broth, chili powder, cumin, oregano, salt, and pepper. Stir well to combine.
4. Reduce the heat to low and let the chili simmer for 30 minutes, stirring occasionally.

Calories: 420   **Protein:** 15g   **Fat:** 5g   **Carbohydrates:** 80g

10.15 Spaghetti Squash with Marinara Sauce and Grilled Vegetables

Preparation time: 15 minutes   **Cooking time:** 45 minutes   **Servings:** 4

Ingredients:

- 1 medium spaghetti squash
- 2 tablespoons olive oil, divided
- 1 onion, finely chopped
- 2 cloves garlic, minced
- 1 can (28 ounces) crushed tomatoes
- 1 teaspoon dried basil

- 1 teaspoon dried oregano
- Salt and pepper to taste
- 1 zucchini, sliced
- 1 bell pepper, sliced
- 1 eggplant, sliced
- Fresh basil (for garnish)

Directions:

For the Spaghetti Squash:

1. Preheat your oven to 400°F (200°C).
2. Cut the spaghetti squash in half lengthwise and scoop out the seeds.
3. Brush the inside of each half with 1 tablespoon of olive oil. Place them cut side down on a baking sheet.
4. Roast for 35-40 minutes, or until the flesh of the squash is easily shredded with a fork.
5. Once cooked, use a fork to scrape out the "spaghetti" strands and set aside.

For the Marinara Sauce:

1. In a saucepan over medium heat, warm the remaining tablespoon of olive oil.
2. Add the chopped onion and garlic, and sauté until translucent.
3. Stir in the crushed tomatoes, dried basil, dried oregano, salt, and pepper. Bring to a simmer and let cook for 15-20 minutes.

For the Grilled Vegetables:

1. Preheat a grill or grill pan over medium-high heat.
2. Brush the zucchini, bell pepper, and eggplant slices with a bit of olive oil and season with salt and pepper.
3. Grill each vegetable for 3-4 minutes on each side or until they have nice grill marks and are tender.

To serve, divide the spaghetti squash strands among the plates, top with marinara sauce, grilled vegetables, and garnish with fresh basil.

Calories: 210   **Protein:** 5g   **Fat:** 7g   **Carbohydrates:** 38g

11 Soup and Stew Recipes

11.1 Lentil and Vegetable Soup

Preparation time: 15 minutes   **Cooking time:** 45 minutes   **Servings:** 6

Ingredients:

- 2 tablespoons olive oil
- 1 large onion, chopped
- 2 cloves garlic, minced
- 2 carrots, diced
- 2 celery stalks, diced
- 1 cup dried lentils, rinsed and sorted
- 1 teaspoon dried thyme
- 1 teaspoon dried oregano
- 1 can (14.5 ounces) diced tomatoes
- 6 cups low-sodium vegetable broth
- Salt and pepper to taste
- 2 cups chopped spinach or kale

Directions:

1. In a large pot, heat the olive oil over medium heat. Add the onion and garlic and sauté until the onion is translucent, about 5 minutes.
2. Add the carrots, celery, lentils, thyme, and oregano. Stir until the lentils are well coated in the oil.
3. Add the diced tomatoes and vegetable broth. Bring the mixture to a boil, then reduce the heat and simmer, covered, for about 30-35 minutes, until the lentils are tender.
4. Season the soup with salt and pepper. Stir in the chopped spinach or kale and continue to cook just until the greens are wilted.
5. Serve the soup hot, with whole grain bread if desired.

Calories: 210   **Protein:** 11g   **Fat:** 7g   **Carbohydrates:** 29g

11.2 Hearty Vegetable and Barley Soup

Preparation time: 20 minutes   **Cooking time:** 60 minutes   **Servings:** 6

Ingredients:

- 1 tablespoon olive oil
- 1 large onion, chopped
- 2 cloves garlic, minced
- 2 carrots, peeled and chopped
- 2 celery stalks, chopped
- 1 cup chopped green beans
- 1 red bell pepper, chopped
- 1/2 cup pearl barley
- 1 teaspoon dried thyme
- 1 can (14.5 ounces) diced tomatoes
- 6 cups low-sodium vegetable broth
- Salt and pepper to taste
- 2 cups chopped kale

Directions:

1. In a large pot, heat the olive oil over medium heat. Add the onion and garlic, and sauté until the onion is translucent, about 5 minutes.
2. Add the carrots, celery, green beans, bell pepper, barley, and thyme. Stir for a few minutes until the vegetables begin to soften.
3. Add the diced tomatoes and vegetable broth. Bring the soup to a boil.
4. Reduce the heat to low and let it simmer, covered, for about 50-60 minutes, or until the barley is tender.
5. Season the soup with salt and pepper. Stir in the kale and cook for an additional 5 minutes, until the kale is wilted.
6. Serve the soup hot, perhaps with a side of whole grain bread.

Calories: 180   **Protein:** 5g   **Fat:** 3g   **Carbohydrates:** 33g

11.3 Tomato Basil Soup with Whole Grain Croutons

Preparation time: 15 minutes   **Cooking time:** 30 minutes   **Servings:** 6

Ingredients:

- 2 tablespoons olive oil
- 1 large onion, chopped
- 4 cloves garlic, minced
- 2 cans (28 ounces each) diced tomatoes
- 3 cups vegetable broth
- 1/2 cup chopped fresh basil
- Salt and pepper to taste
- 1 cup whole grain bread cubes
- Cooking spray

Directions:

1. In a large pot, heat the olive oil over medium heat. Add the onion and garlic, and sauté until the onion is translucent, about 5 minutes.
2. Add the diced tomatoes (with juice) and vegetable broth. Bring to a boil, then reduce heat and simmer for 20 minutes.
3. In the meantime, preheat oven to 375 degrees F (190 degrees C). Arrange bread cubes on a baking sheet and lightly coat with cooking spray. Bake until toasted, about 10-15 minutes.
4. Add the basil to the soup and use an immersion blender to puree the soup until smooth. If you don't have an immersion blender, you can transfer the soup in batches to a countertop blender.
5. Season the soup with salt and pepper to taste. Serve hot with whole grain croutons on top.

Calories: 190   **Protein:** 6g   **Fat:** 6g   **Carbohydrates:** 29g

11.4 Quinoa, Kale, and Chickpea Soup

Preparation time: 15 minutes   **Cooking time:** 25 minutes   **Servings:** 6

Ingredients:

- 1 tablespoon olive oil
- 1 medium onion, chopped
- 3 cloves garlic, minced
- 1 teaspoon cumin
- 1 cup quinoa, rinsed
- 1 can (15 ounces) chickpeas, rinsed and drained
- 1 can (14.5 ounces) diced tomatoes
- 6 cups vegetable broth
- 4 cups chopped kale
- Salt and pepper to taste
- Juice of 1 lemon

Directions:

1. Heat the olive oil in a large pot over medium heat. Add the onion and garlic and sauté until the onion is translucent, about 5 minutes.
2. Add the cumin and quinoa to the pot and cook for a minute, stirring constantly.
3. Add the chickpeas, diced tomatoes, and vegetable broth to the pot. Bring to a boil, then reduce heat and simmer for 20 minutes, until the quinoa is cooked.
4. Add the kale to the pot and cook for a few more minutes, until the kale is wilted.
5. Season the soup with salt, pepper, and lemon juice to taste. Serve hot.

Calories: 260   **Protein:** 12g   **Fat:** 5g   **Carbohydrates:** 45g

11.5 Mushroom and Wild Rice Soup

Preparation time: 15 minutes   **Cooking time:** 45 minutes   **Servings:** 6

Ingredients:

- 1 tablespoon olive oil
- 1 medium onion, diced
- 2 carrots, diced
- 2 celery stalks, diced
- 2 cloves garlic, minced
- 1 pound assorted mushrooms, sliced
- 1 cup wild rice
- 6 cups vegetable broth
- 1 teaspoon dried thyme
- Salt and pepper to taste
- Fresh parsley for garnish

Directions:

1. Heat the olive oil in a large pot over medium heat. Add the onion, carrots, and celery and sauté until the vegetables are tender, about 5 minutes.
2. Add the garlic and mushrooms to the pot and continue to sauté until the mushrooms are browned, about 5 minutes.
3. Add the wild rice, vegetable broth, and dried thyme to the pot. Bring to a boil, then reduce heat to low, cover, and simmer for about 35-40 minutes, until the rice is cooked.
4. Season the soup with salt and pepper to taste. Serve hot, garnished with fresh parsley.

Calories: 220   **Protein:** 8g   **Fat:** 4g   **Carbohydrates:** 40g

11.6 Pumpkin and Sweet Potato Soup

Preparation time: 15 minutes   **Cooking time:** 50 minutes   **Servings:** 6

Ingredients:

- 1 tablespoon olive oil
- 1 medium onion, diced
- 2 cloves garlic, minced
- 1 large sweet potato, peeled and cubed
- 2 cups pumpkin puree
- 4 cups vegetable broth
- 1 teaspoon ground cinnamon
- 1/2 teaspoon ground nutmeg
- Salt and pepper to taste
- Pumpkin seeds for garnish (optional)

Directions:

1. Heat the olive oil in a large pot over medium heat. Add the onion and garlic, and sauté until they start to soften, about 5 minutes.
2. Add the cubed sweet potato to the pot and continue to cook for another 5 minutes, until it starts to soften.
3. Add the pumpkin puree, vegetable broth, ground cinnamon, and ground nutmeg to the pot. Bring the mixture to a boil, then reduce heat to low and let it simmer for about 30-40 minutes, until the sweet potato is completely soft.
4. Using an immersion blender, blend the soup until smooth. If you don't have an immersion blender, you can also carefully transfer the soup to a regular blender in batches and blend until smooth.
5. Season the soup with salt and pepper to taste. Serve hot, garnished with pumpkin seeds, if desired.

Calories: 130   **Protein:** 3g   **Fat:** 2.5g   **Carbohydrates:** 27g

11.7 Butternut Squash and Apple Soup

Preparation time: 20 minutes   **Cooking time:** 45 minutes   **Servings:** 6

Ingredients:

- 1 medium butternut squash, peeled and diced
- 2 medium apples, peeled, cored, and chopped
- 1 medium onion, chopped
- 2 cloves garlic, minced
- 4 cups vegetable broth
- 1 teaspoon ground cinnamon
- 1/4 teaspoon ground nutmeg
- 1 tablespoon olive oil
- Salt and pepper to taste
- Pumpkin seeds for garnish (optional)

Directions:

1. Heat the olive oil in a large pot over medium heat. Add the onion and garlic, and sauté until they start to soften, about 5 minutes.
2. Add the diced butternut squash, chopped apples, ground cinnamon, and nutmeg to the pot. Sauté for another 5 minutes, until the squash and apples start to soften.
3. Add the vegetable broth to the pot and bring the mixture to a boil. Once boiling, reduce the heat to low and let the soup simmer for about 30-35 minutes, until the squash and apples are completely soft.
4. Using an immersion blender, blend the soup until smooth. If you don't have an immersion blender, you can also carefully transfer the soup to a regular blender in batches and blend until smooth.
5. Season the soup with salt and pepper to taste. Serve hot, garnished with pumpkin seeds, if desired.

Calories: 140   **Protein:** 2g   **Fat:** 2g   **Carbohydrates:** 33g

11.8 Chicken, Brown Rice, and Vegetable Soup

Preparation time: 20 minutes   **Cooking time:** 50 minutes   **Servings:** 6

Ingredients:

- 1 cup brown rice, uncooked
- 1 lb chicken breast, cubed
- 1 medium onion, diced
- 2 carrots, peeled and chopped
- 2 celery stalks, chopped
- 1 bell pepper, chopped
- 1 zucchini, chopped
- 4 cloves of garlic, minced
- 1 tablespoon olive oil
- 6 cups chicken broth
- 1 teaspoon dried thyme
- 1 teaspoon dried oregano
- Salt and pepper to taste
- Fresh parsley for garnish (optional)

Directions:

1. In a large pot, heat the olive oil over medium heat. Add the onion, carrots, and celery, and sauté for about 5 minutes, until the onions become translucent.
2. Add the garlic and chicken to the pot. Continue to cook until the chicken is browned on all sides.
3. Add the bell pepper, zucchini, dried thyme, and oregano to the pot. Sauté for another couple of minutes.
4. Add the uncooked brown rice to the pot, and stir everything together.
5. Pour in the chicken broth, and bring the soup to a simmer. Cover and let it simmer for about 35-40 minutes, or until the rice is cooked and the vegetables are tender.
6. Season the soup with salt and pepper to taste. Serve hot, garnished with fresh parsley if desired.

Calories: 230   **Protein:** 20g   **Fat:** 5g   **Carbohydrates:** 25g

11.9 Spicy Black Bean and Corn Soup

Preparation time: 15 minutes   **Cooking time:** 30 minutes   **Servings:** 6

Ingredients:

- 2 cans (15 oz each) black beans, drained and rinsed
- 1 can (15 oz) sweet corn, drained
- 1 medium onion, chopped
- 3 cloves of garlic, minced
- 1 jalapeno pepper, seeded and finely chopped
- 1 red bell pepper, chopped
- 1 can (14.5 oz) diced tomatoes
- 4 cups vegetable broth
- 1 teaspoon ground cumin
- 1/2 teaspoon chili powder
- Salt and pepper to taste
- 2 tablespoons olive oil
- Fresh cilantro for garnish (optional)
- Lime wedges for serving (optional)

Directions:

1. In a large pot, heat the olive oil over medium heat. Add the onion, garlic, jalapeno, and bell pepper. Cook for about 5 minutes, until the vegetables are softened.
2. Stir in the cumin and chili powder. Cook for another minute, until the spices are fragrant.
3. Add the black beans, corn, diced tomatoes, and vegetable broth to the pot. Stir everything together, and bring the soup to a simmer.
4. Reduce the heat to low, cover the pot, and let it simmer for about 20 minutes, so that the flavors can meld together.
5. Season the soup with salt and pepper to taste. If you like a smoother texture, you can use an immersion blender to partially puree the soup, leaving some chunks for texture.
6. Serve hot, garnished with fresh cilantro and a squeeze of lime if desired.

Calories: 210   **Protein:** 9g   **Fat:** 5g   **Carbohydrates:** 37g

11.10 Moroccan Style Chickpea and Quinoa Stew

Preparation time: 15 minutes   **Cooking time:** 35 minutes   **Servings:** 6

Ingredients:

- 1 tablespoon olive oil
- 1 medium onion, chopped
- 3 cloves garlic, minced
- 2 medium carrots, peeled and diced
- 1 bell pepper, diced
- 2 teaspoons ground cumin
- 1 teaspoon ground coriander
- 1/2 teaspoon ground cinnamon
- 1/2 teaspoon turmeric
- 1/4 teaspoon cayenne pepper (optional, for heat)
- 1 can (15 oz) chickpeas, rinsed and drained
- 1 cup quinoa, rinsed
- 1 can (28 oz) diced tomatoes, with juice
- 4 cups vegetable broth
- Salt and pepper to taste
- Chopped fresh cilantro for garnish

Directions:

1. Heat the olive oil in a large pot over medium heat. Add the onion, garlic, carrots, and bell pepper. Cook for 5-7 minutes until vegetables are softened.
2. Add the cumin, coriander, cinnamon, turmeric, and cayenne pepper (if using). Stir to coat the vegetables in the spices and cook for another minute until fragrant.
3. Add the chickpeas, quinoa, diced tomatoes with their juice, and vegetable broth to the pot. Bring to a boil.
4. Reduce heat to low, cover the pot, and simmer for 25-30 minutes, until the quinoa is cooked and the stew has thickened.
5. Season with salt and pepper to taste. Serve hot, garnished with chopped fresh cilantro.

Calories: 265   **Protein:** 10g   **Fat:** 6g   **Carbohydrates:** 44g

12 Juices, Smoothies, and Healthy Drink Recipes

12.1 Green Detox Juice with Kale and Apples

Preparation time: 10 minutes   **Cooking time:** 0 minutes   **Servings:** 2

Ingredients:

- 2 large green apples, cored
- 6 large kale leaves, washed
- 1 medium-sized cucumber
- 1 medium-sized lemon, peeled
- 1-inch piece of fresh ginger, peeled

Directions:

1. Prepare the fruits and vegetables by washing them thoroughly.
2. Core the apples, peel the lemon and ginger, and cut the cucumber into smaller pieces that will fit in your juicer.
3. Run the apples, kale, cucumber, lemon, and ginger through your juicer.
4. Stir the juice to combine and serve immediately. If desired, you can pour it over ice.

Calories: 110   **Protein:** 2.5g   **Fat:** 0.6g   **Carbohydrates:** 27g

12.2 Berry Antioxidant Smoothie

Preparation time: 5 minutes   **Cooking time:** 0 minutes   **Servings:** 2

Ingredients:

- 2 cups of mixed berries (strawberries, blueberries, raspberries)
- 1 banana
- 1 cup of spinach
- 1 cup of almond milk (unsweetened)
- 1 tablespoon of chia seeds

Directions:

1. Prepare the ingredients: wash the mixed berries and spinach thoroughly, peel the banana.
2. Add all the ingredients into a blender.
3. Blend until smooth, adding a little more almond milk if needed.
4. Pour into glasses and serve immediately.

Calories: 150   **Protein:** 4g   **Fat:** 3g   **Carbohydrates:** 28g

12.3 Beetroot and Carrot Liver Cleanse Juice

Preparation time: 10 minutes   **Cooking time:** 0 minutes   **Servings:** 2

Ingredients:

- 1 medium-sized beetroot
- 2 large carrots
- 1 green apple
- 1 piece of fresh ginger (about 1 inch)
- 1 lemon

Directions:

1. Clean all the ingredients thoroughly. Peel the beetroot, carrots, and ginger. Cut the apple into quarters and remove the core.
2. Feed the beetroot, carrots, apple, and ginger through a juicer.
3. Squeeze the juice of the lemon into the mixture.
4. Stir well to combine, then divide the juice between two glasses.
5. Serve immediately for the most health benefits.

Calories: 120   **Protein:** 2g   **Fat:** 1g   **Carbohydrates:** 28g

12.4 Pineapple and Ginger Digestive Smoothie

Preparation time: 10 minutes   **Cooking time:** 0 minutes   **Servings:** 2

Ingredients:

- 2 cups fresh pineapple chunks
- 1 cup unsweetened almond milk
- 1 banana
- 1 tablespoon fresh ginger, peeled and grated
- Ice cubes (optional)

Directions:

1. Add the pineapple chunks, almond milk, banana, and ginger to a blender.
2. Blend on high speed until everything is completely smooth. If desired, add ice cubes and blend again to make the smoothie colder.
3. Divide the smoothie into two glasses and serve immediately.

Calories: 130   **Protein:** 2g   **Fat:** 2g   **Carbohydrates:** 31g

12.5 Turmeric and Lemon Morning Detox Water

Preparation time: 5 minutes   **Cooking time:** 0 minutes   **Servings:** 1

Ingredients:

- 1 cup of warm water
- 1 tablespoon lemon juice
- 1/2 teaspoon turmeric powder
- A pinch of black pepper (to increase turmeric absorption)

Directions:

1. Warm the water until it reaches a comfortable temperature to drink.
2. Stir in the lemon juice, turmeric powder, and a pinch of black pepper.
3. Consume immediately, preferably first thing in the morning on an empty stomach.

Calories: 10   **Protein:** 0.2g   **Fat:** 0.1g   **Carbohydrates:** 2g

12.6 Apple Cider Vinegar and Honey Weight Loss Drink

Preparation time: 5 minutes   **Cooking time:** 0 minutes   **Servings:** 1

Ingredients:

- 1 cup of warm water
- 2 tablespoons of apple cider vinegar
- 1 tablespoon of raw honey

Directions:

1. Warm the water until it reaches a comfortable temperature to drink.
2. Stir in the apple cider vinegar and raw honey until fully dissolved.
3. Consume this mixture once a day, preferably in the morning on an empty stomach.

Calories: 65   **Protein:** 0g   **Fat:** 0g   **Carbohydrates:** 17g

12.7 Spinach, Cucumber, and Celery Hydration Juice

Preparation time: 10 minutes   **Cooking time:** 0 minutes   **Servings:** 1

Ingredients:

- 2 cups of fresh spinach
- 1 large cucumber
- 2 celery stalks

Directions:

1. Wash all the vegetables thoroughly.
2. Cut the cucumber and celery into pieces that will fit in your juicer.
3. Start the juicer, then add the spinach, cucumber, and celery in that order.
4. Once all the vegetables have been juiced, stir the mixture and pour it into a glass.
5. Consume immediately for maximum nutrient retention.

Calories: 70   **Protein:** 3g   **Fat:** 0g   **Carbohydrates:** 16g

12.8 Banana, Almond Milk, and Oat Breakfast Smoothie

Preparation time: 5 minutes   **Cooking time:** 0 minutes   **Servings:** 1

Ingredients:

- 1 ripe banana
- 1 cup unsweetened almond milk
- 1/4 cup rolled oats
- 1 teaspoon honey (optional)

Directions:

1. Place the banana, almond milk, and rolled oats in a blender.
2. Blend until smooth and all the oats have been completely blended. If desired, add honey for additional sweetness.
3. Pour into a glass and serve immediately.

Calories: 235   **Protein:** 6g   **Fat:** 5g   **Carbohydrates:** 45g

12.9 Pomegranate and Orange Immunity Booster Juice

Preparation time: 10 minutes   **Cooking time:** 0 minutes   **Servings:** 2

Ingredients:

- 2 large pomegranates
- 2 large oranges
- Ice cubes (optional)

Directions:

1. Cut the pomegranates in half. Hold each half over a large bowl, cut side down, and tap the back with a wooden spoon to release the seeds (also known as arils). Do this for all 4 halves.
2. Transfer the seeds to a juice press or a juicer and extract the juice. Strain the juice to remove any leftover particles, if necessary.
3. Cut the oranges in half and squeeze the juice into the same bowl as the pomegranate juice.
4. Stir the juices together until well mixed. If desired, chill the juice in the fridge or serve over ice.

Calories: 130   **Protein:** 2g   **Fat:** 1g   **Carbohydrates:** 31g

12.10   Matcha Green Tea and Spinach Energy Drink

Preparation time: 5 minutes   **Cooking time:** 0 minutes   **Servings:** 2

Ingredients:

- 2 cups of fresh spinach
- 1 teaspoon of matcha green tea powder
- 2 cups of unsweetened almond milk
- 1 ripe banana
- 1 tablespoon of honey or a natural sweetener of choice (optional)

Directions:

1. In a blender, combine the spinach, matcha green tea powder, almond milk, and banana.
2. Blend on high speed until the mixture is completely smooth and creamy, about 1-2 minutes.
3. Taste the drink and if needed, add honey or your preferred sweetener and blend again until mixed.
4. Pour the energy drink into two glasses and serve immediately.

Calories: 115   **Protein:** 3g   **Fat:** 3g   **Carbohydrates:** 20g

13 Healthy Desserts

13.1 Baked Apples with Cinnamon and Walnuts

Preparation time: 15 minutes   **Cooking time:** 30 minutes   **Servings:** 4

Ingredients:

- 4 medium apples
- 1/2 cup chopped walnuts
- 1/4 cup honey
- 1 teaspoon ground cinnamon
- A pinch of nutmeg
- 1/2 cup water

Directions:

1. Preheat your oven to 350°F (175°C).
2. Core the apples, making sure not to cut through the bottom. Create a well about an inch wide.
3. In a small bowl, combine the chopped walnuts, honey, cinnamon, and nutmeg. Stir until well combined.
4. Fill each apple with the walnut mixture, packing it tightly.
5. Place the apples in a baking dish, and pour the water into the bottom of the dish.
6. Bake for 30-35 minutes, or until the apples are cooked through and tender.
7. Allow to cool for a few minutes before serving.

Calories: 240   **Protein:** 3g   **Fat:** 10g   **Carbohydrates:** 40g

13.2 Mixed Berry and Chia Seed Pudding

Preparation time: 10 minutes   **Cooking time:** No cooking required   **Servings:** 4

Ingredients:

- 2 cups of unsweetened almond milk or coconut milk
- 1/2 cup of chia seeds
- 1-2 tablespoons of honey or pure maple syrup (optional)
- 1 teaspoon of vanilla extract
- 2 cups of mixed berries (strawberries, blueberries, raspberries, etc.)

Directions:

1. In a bowl, mix together the almond milk (or coconut milk), chia seeds, sweetener if using, and vanilla extract.
2. Stir well to ensure the chia seeds are fully immersed in the liquid. Let it sit for a few minutes and then stir again to break up any clumps of chia seeds.
3. Cover the bowl and refrigerate for at least 2 hours or overnight until the mixture achieves a pudding-like consistency.
4. When ready to serve, give the pudding a good stir, then portion into bowls and top with a generous helping of mixed berries.

Calories: 220   **Protein:** 7g   **Fat:** 11g   **Carbohydrates:** 24g

13.3 Almond and Date Energy Balls

Preparation time: 15 minutes   **Cooking time:** No cooking required   **Servings:** 12

Ingredients:

- 1 cup almonds
- 1.5 cups pitted dates
- 1 teaspoon vanilla extract
- 1/2 teaspoon cinnamon
- 1/4 teaspoon sea salt
- 2 tablespoons unsweetened shredded coconut for coating (optional)

Directions:

1. Place the almonds in a food processor and pulse until they are finely chopped.
2. Add the pitted dates, vanilla extract, cinnamon, and sea salt. Continue to pulse until the mixture starts to come together.
3. Using your hands, roll the mixture into small balls, about 1 inch in diameter. If desired, roll the energy balls in the shredded coconut to coat them.
4. Place the energy balls in the refrigerator for at least 30 minutes to allow them to firm up before serving.

Calories: 100   **Protein:** 2g   **Fat:** 5g   **Carbohydrates:** 12g

13.4 Greek Yogurt with Honey and Fresh Berries

Preparation time: 5 minutes   **Cooking time:** No cooking required   **Servings:** 1

Ingredients:

- 1 cup non-fat Greek yogurt
- 1 tablespoon honey
- 1/2 cup mixed fresh berries (such as strawberries, blueberries, and raspberries)

Directions:

1. Place the Greek yogurt in a bowl.
2. Drizzle the honey over the Greek yogurt.
3. Top with the fresh berries.
4. Enjoy immediately, or refrigerate for up to one day before eating.

Calories: 180   **Protein:** 20g   **Fat:** 0g   **Carbohydrates:** 28g

13.5 Dark Chocolate Avocado Mousse

Preparation time: 10 minutes   **Cooking time:** No cooking required   **Servings:** 2

Ingredients:

- 1 ripe avocado
- 1/4 cup unsweetened dark cocoa powder
- 3-4 tablespoons honey or a sweetener of your choice
- 1/2 teaspoon pure vanilla extract
- A pinch of sea salt
- Fresh berries for topping (optional)

Directions:

1. Cut the avocado in half, remove the pit, and scoop out the flesh.
2. In a blender or food processor, combine the avocado, cocoa powder, honey, vanilla extract, and a pinch of salt.
3. Blend until smooth, scraping down the sides of the bowl as needed.
4. Taste and adjust the sweetness if needed.
5. Divide the mousse between two serving dishes and refrigerate for at least an hour before serving.
6. Top with fresh berries if desired, and serve.

Calories: 230   **Protein:** 4g   **Fat:** 15g   **Carbohydrates:** 27g

13.6 Healthy Banana Bread with Oats and Honey

Preparation time: 15 minutes   **Cooking time:** 55 minutes   **Servings:** 12

Ingredients:

- 1 1/2 cups mashed bananas (about 3-4 ripe bananas)
- 1/3 cup honey or maple syrup
- 1/2 cup unsweetened almond milk (or milk of your choice)
- 1 teaspoon pure vanilla extract
- 2 eggs
- 1/4 cup unsweetened applesauce
- 1 3/4 cups whole wheat flour
- 1/2 cup rolled oats
- 1 teaspoon baking soda
- 1/2 teaspoon salt
- 1/2 teaspoon cinnamon

Directions:

1. Preheat the oven to 350°F (175°C) and grease a 9x5 inch loaf pan.
2. In a large bowl, mash the bananas. Add the honey, milk, vanilla, eggs, and applesauce, and whisk to combine.
3. In a separate bowl, combine the flour, oats, baking soda, salt, and cinnamon.
4. Gradually add the dry ingredients to the banana mixture, stirring until just combined.
5. Pour the batter into the prepared loaf pan and smooth the top.
6. Bake for 50-60 minutes, or until a toothpick inserted into the center comes out clean. If the top begins to brown too quickly, you can cover it with aluminum foil.
7. Let the bread cool in the pan for 10 minutes, then transfer to a wire rack to cool completely before slicing.

Calories: 160   **Protein:** 4g   **Fat:** 2g   **Carbohydrates:** 32g

13.7 Peanut Butter and Banana Ice Cream (sugar-free)

Preparation time: 10 minutes   **Cooking time:** 2 hours   **Servings:** 4

Ingredients:

- 4 ripe bananas
- 2 tablespoons natural, unsweetened peanut butter
- Optional: Cinnamon or cocoa powder for topping

Directions:

1. Peel and slice the bananas into small chunks. Place in a freezer-safe bag or container and freeze for at least 2 hours, or until solid.
2. Once the bananas are frozen, place them in a food processor or high-powered blender. Blend until the bananas are crumbly.
3. Add the peanut butter to the blender. Continue to blend until the mixture becomes creamy and smooth. You may need to stop and scrape down the sides of the blender a few times.
4. Serve the ice cream immediately for a soft-serve texture, or transfer it to a lidded container and freeze for an additional hour for a more solid texture.
5. Optional: Sprinkle with a little cinnamon or cocoa powder before serving.

Calories: 145   **Protein:** 4g   **Fat:** 3g   **Carbohydrates:** 30g

13.8 Mango and Coconut Chia Pudding

Preparation time: 15 minutes   **Cooking time:** 4 hours or overnight   **Servings:** 4

Ingredients:

- 1/4 cup chia seeds
- 1 cup light coconut milk
- 1 tablespoon honey or a sweetener of choice
- 1 ripe mango, peeled and pitted
- 1/2 cup unsweetened shredded coconut

Directions:

1. In a medium bowl, combine the chia seeds, coconut milk, and honey. Stir well to combine.
2. Cover the bowl and place it in the refrigerator. Let it sit for at least 4 hours, or overnight, until the chia seeds have absorbed the liquid and the mixture has a pudding-like consistency.
3. Cut the mango into small cubes. If you prefer a smooth pudding, you could also puree the mango in a blender or food processor.
4. Layer the chia pudding and mango in four glasses or jars, starting with a layer of chia pudding, then adding a layer of mango, and so on.
5. Top with the shredded coconut before serving.

Calories: 170   **Protein:** 3g   **Fat:** 10g   **Carbohydrates:** 20g

13.9 Oatmeal and Raisin Cookies (sugar-free)

Preparation time: 15 minutes   **Cooking time:** 15 minutes   **Servings:** 12 cookies

Ingredients:

- 2 cups rolled oats
- 1 cup raisins
- 2 ripe bananas, mashed
- 1/4 cup unsweetened apple sauce
- 1 teaspoon cinnamon
- 1/2 teaspoon baking powder
- Pinch of salt

Directions:

1. Preheat your oven to 350°F (175°C) and line a baking sheet with parchment paper.
2. In a large bowl, combine the mashed bananas, apple sauce, cinnamon, baking powder, and salt.
3. Add the rolled oats and raisins into the mixture and stir until well combined.
4. Scoop out heaping tablespoons of the dough and place them on the prepared baking sheet. Flatten each cookie slightly with the back of a spoon.
5. Bake for 15 minutes, or until the cookies are lightly browned and set.
6. Let the cookies cool on the baking sheet for 5 minutes, then transfer them to a wire rack to cool completely.

Calories: 100   **Protein:** 2g   **Fat:** 1g   **Carbohydrates:** 22g

13.10   Grilled Pineapple with Cinnamon and Honey

Preparation time: 10 minutes   **Cooking time:** 10 minutes   **Servings:** 4 servings

Ingredients:

- 1 pineapple, peeled, cored and cut into rings
- 2 tablespoons honey
- 1 teaspoon cinnamon

Directions:

1. Preheat your grill to medium heat.
2. In a small bowl, mix together the honey and cinnamon.
3. Brush the pineapple rings with the honey and cinnamon mixture.
4. Place the pineapple rings on the grill. Cook for about 4-5 minutes on each side or until you see grill marks.
5. Remove the pineapple rings from the grill and let them cool for a few minutes before serving.

Calories: 110   **Protein:** 1g   **Fat:** 0g   **Carbohydrates:** 29g

14 Comprehensive Meal Plans

14.1 4-Week Meal Plan for Detoxing the Liver

Welcome to what could be a game-changing month for your liver: our 4-Week Meal Plan for Detoxing the Liver. Think of this chapter as your comprehensive guide or even a roadmap. It's structured to gradually cleanse your liver over a month, but it's not just about a quick detox and then back to your old ways. Far from it. The idea here is to give your liver a much-needed break, providing it with the essential nutrients it needs to function at its best and to heal itself.

You see, this plan is geared towards reducing the stress on your liver. It does this by minimizing its contact with toxins that often come from processed foods, alcohol, and unhealthy fats. Instead, imagine your meals being filled with foods that are not just good but good for you—foods packed with antioxidants, fiber, lean proteins, and beneficial fats. These are the types of nutrients that aid your liver in its detoxification process and help in its natural repair mechanisms.

Over the course of these four weeks, you'll be introduced to a variety of liver-boosting foods. We're talking about leafy greens, an assortment of nuts and seeds, luscious berries, invigorating citrus fruits, wholesome grains, and lean meats. As each week passes, you'll find that the menu doesn't just benefit your liver but also excites your palate. Rest assured, this isn't a regimen of bland, uninteresting foods; you'll be dining on meals that are as tasty as they are healthful.

So, what can you expect in the days ahead? Well, we've mapped out each day of each week, covering breakfast, lunch, dinner, and yes, even snacks. It's a step-by-step guide aimed at renewing your liver and, by extension, elevating your overall health and wellness.

That said, it's important to note that this plan isn't a one-size-fits-all approach. Each of us has unique nutritional needs and food preferences. This plan is designed to be flexible. Feel free to tailor it to what feels right for your body. The real goal isn't strict adherence but rather a genuine, long-term change in how you approach your diet and health.

By deciding to embark on this 4-week journey, you're making a commitment, not just to your liver, but to your overall well-being. This can be a transformative time—a time to learn, to understand, and to adopt healthier habits that you will hopefully maintain for a lifetime. We're excited for you, not just to experience this new way of eating, but also to discover the myriad health benefits that will likely come along with it. Cheers to a revitalized liver and a more vibrant you!

Week 1	Breakfast	Lunch	Snack	Dinner
Day 1	Berry Antioxidant Smoothie	Lentil and Vegetable Soup	Almond and Date Energy Balls	Vegan Lentil and Vegetable Loaf
Day 2	Banana, Almond Milk, and Oat Breakfast Smoothie	Greek Salad with Grilled Chicken Breast	Greek Yogurt with Honey and Fresh Berries	Baked Sweet Potato with Vegan Chili
Day 3	Green Detox Juice with Kale and Apples	Tomato Basil Soup with Whole Grain Croutons	Grilled Pineapple with Cinnamon and Honey	Spicy Lentil and Vegetable Curry
Day 4	Beetroot and Carrot Liver Cleanse Juice	Chickpea and Vegetable Stir Fry with Brown Rice	Mixed Berry and Chia Seed Pudding	Quinoa Stuffed Bell Peppers
Day 5	Pineapple and Ginger Digestive Smoothie	Eggplant and Chickpea Stew	Almond and Date Energy Balls	Vegan Sweet Potato and Black Bean Enchiladas
Day 6	Matcha Green Tea and Spinach Energy Drink	Lentil Shepherd's Pie	Greek Yogurt with Honey and Fresh Berries	Mushroom and Spinach Lasagna
Day 7	Berry Antioxidant Smoothie	Cauliflower and Potato Curry	Baked Apples with Cinnamon and Walnuts	Baked Falafel with Tzatziki Sauce

Week 2

Repeat the meals from Week 1. You can swap any lunch or dinner meal with another from a different day. Snacks can also be exchanged as per preference.

Week 3	Breakfast	Lunch	Snack	Dinner
Day 1	Green Detox Juice with Kale and Apples	Tomato Basil Soup with Whole Grain Croutons	Baked Apples with Cinnamon and Walnuts	Vegan Pad Thai with Tofu
Day 2	Beetroot and Carrot Liver Cleanse Juice	Chickpea and Vegetable Stir Fry with Brown Rice	Greek Yogurt with Honey and Fresh Berries	Stuffed Zucchini with Quinoa and Black Beans
Day 3	Pineapple and Ginger Digestive Smoothie	Lentil Shepherd's Pie	Almond and Date Energy Balls	Vegetarian Chili with Whole Grain Cornbread
Day 4	Matcha Green Tea and Spinach Energy Drink	Eggplant and Chickpea Stew	Mixed Berry and Chia Seed Pudding	Spaghetti Squash with Marinara Sauce and Grilled Vegetables
Day 5	Banana, Almond Milk, and Oat Breakfast Smoothie	Greek Salad with Grilled Chicken Breast	Grilled Pineapple with Cinnamon and Honey	Quinoa Stuffed Bell Peppers
Day 6	Berry Antioxidant Smoothie	Lentil and Vegetable Soup	Greek Yogurt with Honey and Fresh Berries	Baked Sweet Potato with Vegan Chili
Day 7	Green Detox Juice with Kale and Apples	Cauliflower and Potato Curry	Almond and Date Energy Balls	Vegan Lentil and Vegetable Loaf

Week 4

Repeat the meals from Week 3. Again, feel free to swap any lunch, dinner, or snack with another from a different day.

Remember to drink plenty of water throughout the day, and make adjustments as needed based on your dietary needs and preferences. This meal plan provides a variety of nutrients from different sources and aims to be both flavorful and satisfying while promoting liver health.

14.2 8-Week Meal Plan for Maintaining Liver Health

Welcome to a brand new chapter in your journey to better health: the 8-Week Meal Plan for Maintaining Liver Health. This is the phase where we keep the momentum going. It's one thing to complete a detox, but what comes after is equally crucial. This 8-week plan is designed with that continuity in mind. It's like the sequel to your 4-week detox plan—similar core principles but with new, mouth-watering recipes to keep your dining experience far from dull.

Why an 8-week plan, you ask? Well, eight weeks gives us ample time not just to maintain the gains your liver has made but also to help you firmly establish healthy eating habits. These are habits you'll hopefully keep long after these two months have passed. It's about building on your successes and making them a permanent part of your life.

You'll find one core idea that we revisit throughout this plan: the importance of variety. Sticking to a meal plan shouldn't feel like a chore, and let's be honest—eating the same thing over and over gets old fast. That's why we've spiced things up a bit, rotating different recipes every week to keep your taste buds interested and to ensure you're getting a well-rounded mix of nutrients. While you'll encounter some familiar favorites from your detox phase, expect to meet some new dishes that will make mealtime something to look forward to.

But let's be clear: this isn't just about following a meal schedule for two months. This plan aspires to be more than a regimen; it aims to shift your whole approach to eating and well-being. By the end of these eight weeks, we hope you'll see this not merely as a diet but as a lifestyle change. One that prioritizes whole foods, considers mindful eating, and recognizes how crucial our dietary choices are to the health of our liver.

That being said, we understand that life happens and flexibility is key. Whether you have unique dietary needs or simply want to switch things around a bit, this plan accommodates that. The principles remain the same, even if the ingredients change. Adapt it to make it work for you.

So, let's get started, shall we? The next eight weeks promise to be a delightful, nourishing, and possibly transformative experience. Your liver, no doubt, will thank you. And who knows? You might just discover a new favorite dish or two along the way. Here's to a sustained and enriching journey towards better liver health!

Week 1 and Week 2 are the same as the 1st and 2nd weeks in the 4-week Detox Plan. You can refer to that.

Week 3	Breakfast	Lunch	Snack	Dinner
Day 1	Matcha Green Tea and Spinach Energy Drink	Hearty Vegetable and Barley Soup	Oatmeal and Raisin Cookies (sugar-free)	Baked Falafel with Tzatziki Sauce
Day 2	Beetroot and Carrot Liver Cleanse Juice	Quinoa, Kale, and Chickpea Soup	Greek Yogurt with Honey and Fresh Berries	Vegan Sweet Potato and Black Bean Enchiladas
Day 3	Banana, Almond Milk, and Oat Breakfast Smoothie	Mushroom and Wild Rice Soup	Baked Apples with Cinnamon and Walnuts	Spaghetti Squash with Marinara Sauce and Grilled Vegetables
Day 4	Pineapple and Ginger Digestive Smoothie	Pumpkin and Sweet Potato Soup	Almond and Date Energy Balls	Vegan Lentil and Vegetable Loaf
Day 5	Green Detox Juice with Kale and Apples	Butternut Squash and Apple Soup	Grilled Pineapple with Cinnamon and Honey	Quinoa Stuffed Bell Peppers
Day 6	Berry Antioxidant Smoothie	Chicken, Brown Rice, and Vegetable Soup	Peanut Butter and Banana Ice Cream (sugar-free)	Vegan Pad Thai with Tofu
Day 7	Beetroot and Carrot Liver Cleanse Juice	Spicy Black Bean and Corn Soup	Healthy Banana Bread with Oats and Honey	Mushroom and Spinach Lasagna

Week 4

Repeat the meals from Week 3.

Week 5 and Week 6

Repeat the meals from Week 1 and 2 to provide a sense of familiarity while still rotating through the wide variety of recipes available.

Week 7	Breakfast	Lunch	Snack	Dinner
Day 1	Green Detox Juice with Kale and Apples	Moroccan Style Chickpea and Quinoa Stew	Almond and Date Energy Balls	Stuffed Zucchini with Quinoa and Black Beans
Day 2	Matcha Green Tea and Spinach Energy Drink	Lentil Shepherd's Pie	Greek Yogurt with Honey and Fresh Berries	Spaghetti Squash with Marinara Sauce and Grilled Vegetables
Day 3	Pineapple and Ginger Digestive Smoothie	Tomato Basil Soup with Whole Grain Croutons	Baked Apples with Cinnamon and Walnuts	Lentil and Vegetable Soup
Day 4	Berry Antioxidant Smoothie	Chickpea and Vegetable Stir Fry with Brown Rice	Peanut Butter and Banana Ice Cream (sugar-free)	Mushroom and Spinach Lasagna
Day 5	Beetroot and Carrot Liver Cleanse Juice	Eggplant and Chickpea Stew	Grilled Pineapple with Cinnamon and Honey	Baked Sweet Potato with Vegan Chili
Day 6	Banana, Almond Milk, and Oat Breakfast Smoothie	Quinoa, Kale, and Chickpea Soup	Healthy Banana Bread with Oats and Honey	Lentil Shepherd's Pie
Day 7	Green Detox Juice with Kale and Apples	Cauliflower and Potato Curry	Almond and Date Energy Balls	Vegan Sweet Potato and Black Bean Enchiladas

Week 8

Repeat the meals from Week 7.

15 The Journey Beyond the Kitchen

15.1 Dealing with Challenges and Staying Motivated

Embarking on a dietary transformation, especially one aimed at tackling something as serious as fatty liver disease, is no walk in the park. It can be tough, and the road may be long. But let's be real—this isn't a sprint; it's more like a marathon. So how do you keep your eyes on the prize when the journey is long and sometimes daunting? Well, I've got some tips that might just make the trip a little easier.

First off, let's talk about pacing yourself. Changing how you eat is a monumental task; it can feel like you're climbing a mountain. But don't stress about conquering it all at once. Start simple. Maybe swap in one or two recipes from this guide into your weekly menu. As you grow accustomed to the new flavors and textures, you can broaden your culinary horizons even further. Take baby steps; Rome wasn't built in a day.

Now, let's tackle goals. Vague ambitions like "losing weight" or "being healthier" might sound good, but they lack the precision that drives action. Try to get a bit more specific with your goals. Instead of aiming to 'eat better,' why not aim to add a vegetable side dish to every dinner this week? Or challenge yourself to try out four new recipes before Sunday rolls around. When you nail these smaller, more achievable goals, you'll feel a surge of satisfaction that keeps the motivational fire burning.

Support is another biggie. It's not just about you and your plate; it's about the network of people around you. Share what you're up to with friends and family. Tell them why it's crucial for you to change your diet. Chances are, they'll be your cheerleaders. They might even join you in munching on that kale salad or sipping that green smoothie. And if your immediate circle isn't enough, tap into the collective wisdom of online communities. Sometimes, knowing that someone else is in the same boat can make all the difference. And hey, life happens. Sometimes you fall off the wagon. You might find yourself diving into a bag of chips or skimping on greens one day. It's okay. Seriously, don't beat yourself up about it. Just look at it as a sort of dietary 'plot twist.' Reflect on what triggered the lapse and figure out how to sidestep it next time. Then, just get back to your routine.

Don't forget to give yourself some well-deserved pats on the back, too. Every little win counts. Relished a new recipe? Score! Opted for a salad when you could have had a cheeseburger? Double score! Celebrate these moments. They're signs that you're making progress, and they make the journey not just endurable but enjoyable.

In essence, you're rewriting your food story here, and that takes time, patience, and a fair bit of resilience. You're bound to face challenges and even stumble a bit. But armed with clear goals, a supportive tribe, and a dash of self-compassion, you're more than equipped to stay the course. Remember, every single choice you make that aligns with your new lifestyle is a win, no matter how trivial it may seem. Keep racking up those small victories, and before you know it, you'll have won your marathon.

15.2 The Role of Regular Check-ups and Monitoring Your Progress

Addressing fatty liver disease isn't merely a matter of changing your diet or increasing your activity level, though both are critical. One of the sneaky things about this condition is that it often flies under the radar, offering few, if any, warning signs, particularly in its initial stages. This makes regular medical check-ups an indispensable part of managing your health.

At the heart of these check-ups are liver function tests. Basically, they're blood tests that look for signs of liver trouble. By measuring specific enzymes and proteins in your bloodstream, these tests provide an initial glimpse into how well your liver is holding up. If those levels are off, it's a red flag. The idea is to keep an eye on these markers over time to see how your liver is responding to changes in your diet, exercise habits, and lifestyle.

Then there's ultrasound imaging. It's a painless procedure that offers a more visual check-up of your liver. Using sound waves, this technique generates images that allow healthcare providers to eyeball your liver's size, texture, and shape. It's especially useful for spotting fat accumulation, one of the defining features of fatty liver disease.

While you're there for your check-up, expect a hands-on physical examination too. Your healthcare provider will be on the lookout for physical signs, like jaundice or fluid buildup in your abdomen. Now, these are often late-stage symptoms, but if they're present, it's a loud and clear signal that more aggressive treatment is needed.

Beyond the liver-centric aspects of your healthcare, these appointments are an excellent opportunity to take stock of other health factors that often go hand-in-hand with fatty liver disease. I'm talking about things like your weight, your blood pressure, your cholesterol, and your blood sugar levels. Each of these can offer insights not only into your liver's health but into your broader wellbeing.

Your medical appointments are also a good time for some honest dialogue with your healthcare provider. Maybe you're struggling with some of the lifestyle changes you need to make. Or perhaps you've got questions or concerns about your treatment plan. Even small victories in your journey can be acknowledged and celebrated here.

In between these visits, you've got an important job: self-monitoring. Essentially, you're tracking the ins and outs of your daily life—from what you're eating and how much you're moving, to how well you're sticking to your medication schedule. This isn't just busy work; it's about becoming more aware of your habits and holding yourself accountable. Plus, it provides some valuable real-time feedback that can help you adjust your course as needed.

In a nutshell, managing fatty liver disease is a marathon, not a sprint. It's a commitment to your long-term health that requires both professional oversight and a healthy dose of personal responsibility. Your medical check-ups give you a detailed roadmap, penned by healthcare experts, while self-monitoring lets you navigate your daily journey. Each reinforces the other, making for a well-rounded approach to keeping this condition in check. And remember, every step forward is progress, no matter how small it might seem at the time.

16 Conclusion

16.1 Staying on Track for a Healthy Liver and a Healthier You

So, here we are, at what seems like the end of our informational journey. But let's be real: this is just your starting point toward a healthier liver and a more fulfilling life. Think of this guide as a sort of "Liver Health 101" textbook; it gives you the foundational elements you need to kickstart lifestyle changes that do your liver—and your whole self—a world of good.

It's easy to think of conquering fatty liver disease as merely a diet plan or a 'foods to avoid' list. But it's actually so much more than that. This journey invites you to redefine your relationship with what's on your plate. Food isn't just comfort or pleasure; it's fuel. It's what powers you to live, to enjoy, to love. A balanced diet brimming with colorful fruits, crisp vegetables, hearty whole grains, and lean meats isn't just a boon for your liver; it's a recipe for a life that feels more, well, alive.

Then, of course, there's exercise. Now, don't let that word scare you off. Exercise isn't just about dropping pounds or building muscles. It's also your ticket to a happier heart, a sunnier disposition, and energy levels that don't bottom out by mid-afternoon. The secret? Finding a form of movement that doesn't feel like a chore. Whether that's a morning jog, an evening swim, a weekend bike ride, or a daily yoga ritual is entirely up to you.

Let's not forget the unsung heroes of health management: regular medical check-ups and self-monitoring. Think of these as your personal health "audit and feedback" system. They help you catch potential problems early, track your progress, and, importantly, they offer little milestones for you to celebrate. This is you taking the reins of your own health—making decisions informed by facts, not fear.

Ah, challenges. There will be bumps on this road; that's almost guaranteed. But remember, setbacks are not roadblocks; they're detours. They're chances to learn, grow, and, dare I say, become a more resilient version of yourself. In short, they're just part of the journey toward health.

Sometimes, though, even detours can feel discouraging, especially if you're navigating them alone. That's why finding a community—either online or in the flesh—can make all the difference. It's reassuring to know that there are others who've been where you are, who know what you're going through, and who can offer the kind of support that only shared experience can provide.

Look, healing isn't a sprint. It's a marathon that you can only finish one step at a time. Every small win, whether it's losing your first pound or forgoing that second helping of dessert, is a cause for celebration. Keep your eyes on the prize: a healthier you, with a liver that's doing its job like a champ.

To wrap it all up, managing fatty liver disease isn't something you tackle with a single strategy. It's more like assembling a puzzle, with pieces that include a nutritious diet, regular physical activity, consistent medical check-ups, ongoing self-monitoring, community support, and heaps of patience. But every piece you place brings you closer to the full picture of health. And every step you take, armed with the knowledge and tools you've gained, is a win. So take that first step, and then the next, knowing you've got what it takes to live a healthier, happier life.

17 Cooking Conversion Guide: From American to International Units (and Vice Versa)

17.1 Dry Measurements

TSP	TBSP	Cup	Fluid Oz	Grams/Pound
3 tsp	1 tbsp	1/16 C	1/2 oz	14 g
6 tsp	2 tbsp	1/8 C	1 oz	28 g
12 tsp	4 tbsp	1/4 C	2 oz	57 g
16 tsp	5tbsp + 1 tsp	1/3 C	2 2/3 oz	76 g
24 tsp	8 tbsp	1/2 C	4 oz	113 g
32 tsp	10 tbsp + 2 tsp	2/3 C	5 1/3 oz	151 g
36 tsp	12 tbsp	3/4 C	6 oz	170 g
48 tsp	16 tbsp	1 C	8 oz	227 g

17.2 Liquid Measurements

Measure	Fluid Oz	TBSP	TSP	Liters/Milliliters
1 gal	4 quarts	256 tbsp	768 tsp	3.8 liters
4 cups	1 quart	64 tbsp	192 tsp	0.95 liters
2 cups	1 pint	32 tbsp	96 tsp	473 ml
1 cup	8 oz	16 tbsp	48 tsp	237 ml
3/4 cup	6 oz	12 tbsp	36 tsp	177 ml
2/3 cup	5 1/3 oz	10 tbsp + 2 tsp	32 tsp	158 ml
1/2 cup	4 oz	8 tbsp	24 tsp	118 ml
1/3 cup	2 2/3 oz	5 tbsp + 1 tsp	16 tsp	79 ml
1/4 cup	2 oz	4 tbsp	12 tsp	59 ml
1/8 cup	1 oz	2 tbsp	6 tsp	30 ml
1/16 cup	½ oz	1 tbsp	3 tsp	15 ml

17.3 Weight Measurement

Grams	Ounces
14 g	1/2 oz
28 g	1 oz
57 g	2 oz
85 g	3 oz
113 g	4 oz
141 g	5 oz
170 g	6 oz
198 g	7 oz
227 g	8 oz
255 g	9 oz
283 g	10 oz
312 g	11 oz
340 g	12 oz
369 g	13 oz
397 g	14 oz
425 g	15 oz
454 g	1 lb

18 Special Bonus: Unlock Your Free Guide

Dear Reader,

Thank you for investing in your liver health by picking up this book. As a token of my appreciation, I've prepared an exclusive guide just for you!

FATTY LIVER SUPPLEMENT GUIDE:
DECODING THE BEST SUPPLEMENTS FOR OPTIMAL LIVER FUNCTION

Confused about which supplements can actually help in reversing or managing fatty liver disease? This guide takes the guesswork out of the equation, offering you researched-based advice on the most effective supplements for maintaining a healthy liver.

How to Access Your Free Guide:
1. **Scan the QR Code Below**
   - Simply use your phone's camera to scan the QR code, and you'll be directed to the download page.

OR

2. **Visit the Link**
   - If you prefer, you can type the following link into your web browser:
   https://oliviagreenleaf.com

Get your hands on this invaluable guide now and take a leap forward in your journey towards a healthier, happier liver!

Wishing you vibrant health, Olivia Greenleaf

Made in the USA
Las Vegas, NV
12 February 2024